The patient's guide to neurosarcoidosis

Denise Sutherland

sutherlandstudios

Published by Sutherland Studios
sutherland-studios.com.au
ABN: 67 766 872 800

PO Box 3849
Weston Creek ACT 2611
AUSTRALIA

ISBN: 978-0-9872152-5-3

National Library of Australia Cataloguing-in-Publication entry
Creator: Sutherland, Denise, author.
Title: The patient's guide to neurosarcoidosis / Denise Sutherland.
ISBN: 9780987215253 (paperback)
Notes: Includes bibliographical references and index.
Subjects: Sarcoidosis. Nervous system--Diseases. Spinal cord--Diseases. Nerves, Peripheral--Diseases. Brain--Diseases.
Dewey Number: 616.9

Disclaimer

This book is written for general educational and informational purposes only. Although it contains information on medical conditions and treatments, it is in no way intended nor otherwise implied to be medical advice.

If you are concerned or have any questions about any of the issues raised in the book, you should consult a registered medical practitioner. The information provided is by no means complete or exhaustive and therefore does not encompass every aspect of the condition, treatments, or related conditions. Medicine is a constantly changing speciality and, whilst any information was considered correct at the time of publishing, we cannot take into account or claim responsibility for changing trends in the stated conditions or treatment or new evidence that becomes available. Any medications, treatments, and advice are only presented here for informative purposes.

Some of this information is based on personal experience and is not a substitute for obtaining professional medical advice. In no way will the author be liable for either directly, indirectly, consequential, exemplary, or any other damages related to your use of the information contained within this book or any references provided.

Contents

Acknowledgements

I am indebted to several people, who helped me create a more readable and accurate book:

Professor Matthew Cook (immunologist) and Professor Christian Lueck (neurologist), both of the Canberra Hospital and ANU Medical School, helped me to better understand the medical aspects of neurosarcoidosis, its diagnosis, and treatment. They reviewed the first three chapters of this book for accuracy, and I am very grateful for their time and help. Any errors that remain are mine alone.

Betsy Miller, Rachael Cottle, Dr Sadaf Hussain and Freja Swogger, provided valuable feedback and edits. My thanks also to Rachael for her study tips in Chapter 5.

And to all the people who submitted their experiences to the book, *thank you*. I am not naming individuals for privacy reasons, but I thank you all from the bottom of my heart for taking the time and effort to put your stories into words, and for being prepared to share them with the world.

And, as ever, deep gratitude to my husband Ralph for his unswerving love and support.

Note to readers

The first instance of words that are in the glossary appear in **bold**. There is a list of abbreviations on page 146, and the glossary starts on page 147.

Introduction

There aren't many books out there about neurosarcoidosis, and most of them are medical tomes written for neurologists, immunologists, and other specialists. This book is for us patients.

In the first part of the book I do my best to decipher what the researchers and doctors are currently thinking about neurosarcoidosis, its diagnosis and treatment. I also go into some strategies that you might find help you cope with living with neurosarcoidosis, and talk about the psychological and social impacts of the disease.

In the second part of the book I've collected together stories from ten neurosarcoidosis patients. I hope that you will find some common ground with some of the other patients here, and not feel so alone. My experiences are included in that section, but to get you started, here is my story.

I think I might have had neurosarcoidosis since around 2003, but it's impossible to know for sure. I didn't get a diagnosis until late 2010.

My early symptoms were niggling little things that never added up to much — sensations of sticky tape stuck on my toes, fatigue, reduced senses of taste and smell, foot pain, and so on. I got a diagnosis of fibromyalgia and/or chronic fatigue at the time. My ANA blood test was positive, but that didn't indicate much.

In late 2005, I developed a sixth nerve palsy — this stopped one eye from moving, so I had extreme double vision. It put me in hospital for a week. However the tests were all inconclusive, so I was discharged without any treatment or diagnosis. It gradually healed over some months. While we can't prove that this was from neurosarcoidosis, it is probable that it was.

In the summers of 2009 and 2010 I had horribly itchy red raised blistery rashes on my lower legs. My GP didn't think I should see a dermatologist, so I just treated them with cortisone cream, and ice packs. However, when I saw her a few years later, my dermatologist did think the lesions looked like they were caused by sarcoidosis (based on photos I had taken at the time).

Things ramped up in September 2010. I woke up one morning with over a third of my vision gone — there were blotches of blankness in my vision, as if I'd been staring at bright lights. I also had numbness down my right arm, and around my mouth.

I saw my optometrist, and was directed to go immediately to hospital! I was admitted to hospital for three weeks, and was the favourite 'interview subject' for all the medical students. My lumbar puncture was positive, and the MRI showed lesions in my brain, around the optic chiasm. They'd narrowed down my diagnosis to multiple sclerosis, vasculitis, or neurosarcoidosis. They finally started me on high doses of prednisolone on the day I was discharged.

Over the next 11 months, I gradually tapered down off the pred, and started on methotrexate, and then azathioprine (both of which upset my liver), and finally mycophenolate mofetil. *Nearly* all of my vision has returned since then.

During 2011 and 2012 I had frequent appointments with specialists of all sorts, and they gradually all came to the conclusion that neurosarc was the most likely diagnosis. Unfortunately I haven't had a tissue biopsy done, and we missed the opportunity with my leg lesions (which haven't reappeared since I've been on immune suppressants), so I don't have a *definitive* tissue diagnosis, but there isn't any doubt about the diagnosis any more.

Where am I now? Well, I still have a very small blind patch in the centre of one eye, annoyingly, which is from scarring in my brain (in the optic tract). My eyes get tired quickly. My vision is generally pretty blurry, and I don't read for pleasure much any more, but I can still work, with enlarged text sizes on screen.

There may well be sarcoidosis in my liver. I'm tapering down on mycophenolate mofetil, and tolerate it pretty well. My MRI is pretty much clear, the lesions seem to be gone for now. I have recently developed some peripheral neuropathy in my hands and feet. My senses of smell and taste still wax and wane.

In late 2013 I developed (probable) Melkersson-Rosenthal syndrome, which affects the lips and facial nerves, causing swelling in the lips — it can sometimes occur in sarcoidosis. It seems to come and go for me, it isn't permanent, and I hope it stays that way!

The writing of this book was delayed by a year, when my brain fog and fatigue were too bad for me to write. A recent major diet change has drastically helped with my brain fog and fatigue (see page 116), and enabled me to finish this book, thankfully.

I expect that at some point I'll have another neurosarc relapse, and more severe symptoms again, and things will continue to wax and wane like this over the years. I am very thankful that I have the relapsing-remitting form of this disease, which is milder.

I can't work outside of the home, but I still manage to run my own business, do some volunteer work, and look after my family, and I stay as active as I can.

I hope this book is helpful to you. Remember, although you are very rare, you're not alone!

Denise

Canberra, Australia
January 2015

1
Neuro-what?

This book is all about neurosarcoidosis, which is not only hard to say (*new–row–sark–oid–osis*), it's also hard to understand. And it's a hard disease to have. In this chapter I explain the basics of 'general' sarcoidosis, and then neurosarcoidosis.

Sarcoidosis

Sarcoidosis is defined as a **systemic granulomatous** disorder of unknown **aetiology**. Huh? Well, this means it is a disorder that causes **granulomas** to form, that affects the body as whole (systemic), and has an unknown cause (aetiology).

What is a granuloma?

A granuloma is a tiny lump of white blood cells, surrounded by a layer of fibrous cells (see Figure 1 on the next page). White blood cells defend our bodies against invading organisms and foreign objects. White cells are also called **leucocytes**, and there are many types of them. There are a variety of different sorts of white blood cells that can be found inside the granulomas.

> The name leucocyte ('loo-ko-cite') comes from Greek. *Leuko* means 'white', and *kytos* means 'hollow vessel'. *Cyte* means 'cell'.

Fibroblasts are cells that form the outer layer of the granuloma. They are cells usually found in connective tissue that produces **collagen** and other fibres.

1

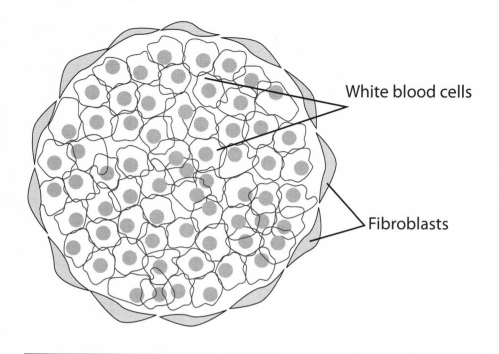

White blood cells

Fibroblasts

Figure 1 — A granuloma

The cells in sarcoidosis granulomas are alive, so they are called **non-necrotising**, or **non-caseating**. These terms just mean that the cells in the granulomas aren't dead. Non-necrotising granulomas are not caused by an infection.

Caseation is when dead cells and diseased tissue turns into a soft cheese-like substance (the name comes from the Latin word for cheese, *caseus*). It is typically a feature of tuberculosis granulomas, which *are* caseating, and are caused by infection.

How do granulomas form?

'**Antigen**' is a general word for any substance that provokes an immune or inflammatory response in the body. Antigens can be produced by the body itself (such as dead cells), or they can come in from outside of the body (viruses, toxins, dust, bacteria and so on).

2

Granulomas are a sign of an abnormal immune response by the body to an antigen. The body keeps trying over and over to get rid of the antigen, but it's unable to break it down or get rid of it, and the lumps of white blood cells around the antigen get bigger, and then remain.

Sarcoidosis granulomas can form anywhere in the body, from the bones to the brain. They can also clump together, forming bigger lumps.

Some other diseases that have granulomas form are **tuberculosis**, **leprosy** (Hansen's disease), **Crohn's disease**, **rheumatoid arthritis**, **histoplasmosis**, **cat-scratch disease**, and some forms of **vasculitis**.

What causes sarcoidosis?

No-one knows the cause of sarcoidosis for sure — yet.

Many immune system disorders result in abnormal inflammation. Inflammatory disorders are the basis of a great deal of disease. Inflammation is the response of body tissues to irritation or injury. Typical inflammatory responses include pain, swelling, redness, and heat.

This sort of chronic inflammation can lead to diseases such as allergies, asthma, rheumatoid arthritis, vasculitis, and sarcoidosis.

The current (still vague) theory about how sarcoidosis develops is:

1. Some people have a genetic predisposition to developing sarcoidosis.
2. They come into contact with certain environmental 'triggers', possibly airborne particles or bacteria (antigens).
3. The body reacts abnormally to these particles, forming granulomas, and sarcoidosis then develops.

Some specific genes have been identified that appear to be associated with sarcoidosis, which may mean that some people are more prone to developing the disease[3].

3

The environmental antigens that seem to trigger sarcoidosis might be microscopic airborne particles, or maybe some bacteria. Bacteria from the **mycobacterium** genus can cause the body to form granulomas, so medical researchers have looked very closely at them in relation to sarcoidosis. Quite a few studies show that mycobacterium genetic material is found in more than half of sarcoidosis patients' granulomas[9,10].

However, mycobacteria are present *everywhere* in our environment, and there are many types of them. It is not yet clear what the presence of these mycobacterial fragments means — it *is not* accurate to say that these bacteria cause the disease.

So, the body identifies these alien intruders (the antigens) and attacks them, as it should. But, instead of the *usual* immune response, which should stop after the antigens have been dealt with, the immune response keeps going.

In the case of sarcoidsosis, the body keeps making white blood cells to attack the intruders, is unable to break them down, and then forms little covered lumps of these cells (the granulomas). As your white blood cells can go anywhere in your body, the granulomas can also form anywhere in your body.

Several studies have shown higher rates of sarcoidosis in people who have frequent exposure to:

- mould, mildew, and musty smells
- high humidity
- smoke
- tree pollen
- agricultural chemicals and pesticides[7]

Metalworkers, firefighters, people who handle building supplies a lot, and those working in the U.S. Navy have higher rates of sarcoidosis than the general population in the USA[3,7].

These environmental associations have led to the suspicion that sarcoidosis is at least in part an abnormal immune response to environmental antigens. But not *all* patients fall into these categories, so this clearly isn't the whole story.

Recent research suggests that **tumor necrosis factor (TNF,** also called **cachexin** or **cachectin)** may be implicated in the development of sarcoidosis granulomas. It is an **adipokine** — a cytokine (cell signaling molecule) secreted by fat cells (**adipocytes**). It is produced by **macrophages** (white blood cells that remove dead cells and pathogens), and some other cells. Its main role is regulating immune cells, and promoting the inflammatory response. When things go wrong with this system, TNF can be implicated in many inflammatory diseases such as rheumatoid arthritis and sarcoidosis[27].

It is reasonable to believe that the development of sarcoidosis is probably the end result of an abnormal immune response to various common environmental triggers, but as you can see the exact cause is not understood yet.

Vitamin D, which acts as both a hormone and a vitamin in our bodies, often occurs in abnormal levels in sarcoidosis patients. Macrophages inside the granulomas convert vitamin D into its active hormonal form, **calcitriol**, leading to abnormally high levels in some patients. These high calcitriol levels can raise calcium levels in the blood (**hypercalcaemia**), and are implicated in immune system dysfunction[27]. Other sarcoidosis patients, however, may have low levels of vitamin D and require supplements.

Who gets sarcoidosis?

Sarcoidosis is most common in people aged 20–40, although it can affect people of any age, including children. Both men and women can get sarcoidosis, but it does appear that more women tend to get it[1]. Scandinavians and black Americans have the highest rates in the world[1]. It seems that sarcoidosis is relatively rare in Asian populations[2.]

How many people get sarcoidosis?

Sarcoidosis occurs throughout the world.

Prevalence rates are often expressed as a ratio, for example '50 patients per 100,000'. In this instance, this means that if you took a group of 100,000 people, 50 people will have that particular condition, on average.

Overall, the average rate for sarcoidosis seems to be roughly 20 cases per 100,000. It is hard to be entirely sure, though, as many cases of sarcoidosis don't have symptoms, so those people are rarely diagnosed with it. Sometimes people only find out they have it by accident, when having a chest x-ray for something else. Sometimes sarcoidosis is only discovered on autopsy.

Some worldwide prevalence rates for sarcoidosis are:

Scandinavians : 5–64 per 100,000, although one study using autopsy results found a rate of 640 per 100,000 in Swedish people[11]

African Americans : 35.5 per 100,000

Caucasian Americans : 10.9 per 100,000

Australians : 4.4–6.3 per 100,000[4]

Japanese : 1–2 per 100,000

Koreans : 0.13 per 100,000

One study has shown the siblings and parents of people with sarcoidosis are up to five times more likely to develop sarcoidosis too, than the regular population[3]. Although parents and siblings are at increased risk, according to this study, the risk is still very low — going roughly from 20 in 100,000 to 100 in 100,000.

Sarcoidosis can occur in children, but is very rare, with a prevalence of less than 1 in 100,000.

What parts of the body can sarcoidosis affect?

Sarcoidosis can affect virtually any part of the body. It most commonly affects the lungs. More than 90% of sarcoidosis patients have it in their lungs, and a high number have it in their lymph nodes (**lymphadenopathy**).

Liver, spleen, skin, and eye involvement are quite common. Sarcoidosis can also affect the nervous system (neurosarcoidosis), heart, pancreas, salivary glands, skeletal muscle, bones, and the upper airway, although these locations are much rarer. Kidney involvement is very rare.

What sort of symptoms do people get?

These are some of the more common symptoms of 'general' sarcoidosis[3]:

- fatigue
- night sweats
- weight loss
- dry cough
- laboured breathing
- chest pain
- coughing up blood
- arthritis
- skin changes, lesions
- sore reddish bumps on the skin
- tender and/or swollen lymph nodes
- inflammation of the coloured part of the eye (**uveitis**)

Prognosis

More than half of people with 'general' sarcoidosis will get better within a few years, and may not even need treatment. And even more (2/3 of the total) will go into remission within 10 years. Remission in this case means that the disease is no longer active.

However, up to a third of patients develop **chronic** sarcoidosis, with more serious problems[3]. Neurosarcoidosis patients fall into this last, less pleasant, category.

The death rate from 'general' sarcoidosis is about 5%. 95% of patients survive.

Neurosarcoidosis

Neurosarcoidosis (neurosarc or NS for short) is the name for sarcoidosis granulomas that form within the **central nervous system** (brain and spinal cord) and/or the **peripheral nervous system** (these are the nerves throughout the rest of the body, outside of the central nervous system).

How many people have it?

From various studies, it seems that patients who have symptoms from neurosarc are roughly 5–13% of the sarcoidosis population[6].

So, using the average rate of 20 per 100,000 for 'general' sarcoidosis, this gives us an average in the general population of 1–2.6 per 100,000 for neurosarcoidosis (see Figure 2 on the next page).

But whatever the exact rate, it's low, and you're officially rare!

It is difficult to pin down exact prevalence rates for neurosarc for a few reasons. Some sarcoidosis patients are discovered (after death) to have had sarcoidosis in their central nervous system, but never had symptoms from it. And to further confuse things, quite a few sarcoidosis patients have neurological symptoms that are *not* caused by NS.

It seems that less than 1% of sarcoidosis patients have *only* neurosarc, and no other evidence of sarcoidosis anywhere else in their bodies. In other words, if you have NS, it is *most* likely that you will have sarcoidosis affecting other parts of your body, such as the lungs, skin, or eyes, as well[1].

Children with neurosarcoidosis tend to have different symptoms from adults with the disease. They have a higher rate of seizures and a low level of cranial nerve involvement, compared to adults[1].

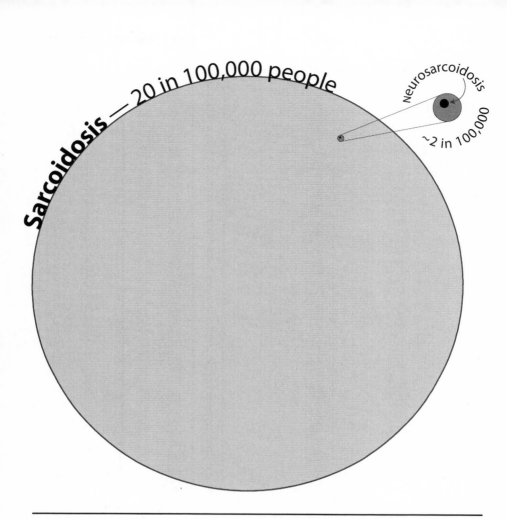

Figure 2 — Prevalence of neurosarcoidosis. The large grey circle represents 100,000 people. The grey dot is people with sarcoidosis. The black dot inside the grey dot is the number with neurosarcoidosis.

As a comparison, the prevalence rate for **multiple sclerosis** ranges between 2–150 per 100,000 (depending on which country you look at), and the prevalence of **lupus** is 20–150 per 100,000.

Neurosarcoidosis symptoms

There are many possible symptoms of neurosarcoidosis, depending on which parts of the central or peripheral nervous system have been affected. The following list goes by major area affected first, and then in order of how common symptoms are.

The brain

Parenchymal brain disease

The **parenchyma** of the brain is the 'grey matter' of the brain, all the functional nervous tissue of the brain. It does not include the connective tissues, blood vessels, and so on (which are called the **stroma**). The brain is affected in about half of neurosarcoidosis patients[28]. The most common areas affected are the **hypothalamus** and **pituitary gland**.

The hypothalamus is an area of the brain that coordinates the **autonomic nervous system**, and the pituitary gland. It secretes hormones that affect the nervous system, such as **dopamine**, and controls body temperature, hunger, thirst, sleep, fatigue, and **circadian rhythms**.

The pituitary gland is located at the base of the hypothalamus. It releases many hormones, including **oxytocin**, and hormones that help with regulating blood pressure, growth, metabolism, sexual organ functions, the thyroid gland and much more.

Problems caused by neurosarcoidosis in these areas of the brain include thyroid disorders, sexual dysfunction, unusual thirst, seizures, and disorders of appetite, libido, temperature control, weight regulation, and sleep.

Eyesight is often affected too, when sarcoidosis granulomas form in the brain. There may be areas of partial changes or vision loss in the field of vision (**scotomas**).

Generally just one of the optic nerves is involved, but sometimes both optic nerves, the **optic chiasm** (where the two optic nerves join in the brain), optic tract, or other areas of the brain associated with vision are damaged. The optic chiasm is typically damaged when the pituitary gland becomes inflamed from sarcoidosis, as it runs around the pituitary gland.

Neuropsychiatric symptoms

Patients with extensive involvement of their brain or spinal cord can sometimes develop psychiatric problems such as depression, poor concentration, **delusions**, dementia, **psychosis**, and hallucinations. These symptoms have been reported in around 20% of NS patients[7,8]. One neurologist at the Cleveland Clinic has said that some level of personality change is normal with neurosarc patients. This is most likely if the frontal lobes are affected by NS.

Personality and mood changes can also be caused by medication, especially corticosteroids (see page 42). And the stress of living with neurosarcoidosis can easily cause depression, too (see Chapter 4).

Seizures

A seizure can be the first manifestation of NS for some patients. A seizure, or convulsion, occurs when the brain sends out abnormal electrical signals to the body. This changes way body functions for a short time. They are different from person to person.

A seizure can cause loss of consciousness, loss of memory, uncontrolled muscle spasms, clenching of teeth, drooling, sudden falling over, and other symptoms. About 15–20% of NS patients develop seizures[6,8]. Any type of seizure can occur (partial, petit mal, tonic clonic and so on)[5]. These can be treated and managed with anticonvulsive drugs, but the underlying neurosarcoidosis also needs to be treated[28].

Hydrocephalus

This rare symptom of neurosarcoidosis is fluid on the brain. The fluid around your brain is there to act as a cushion. However, if too much fluid builds up, it puts pressure on your brain, which isn't a good thing. It can cause memory impairment, sleepiness, and dementia, amongst other serious problems. It requires urgent medical treatment.

Symptoms of hydrocephalus include:

- headache
- vomiting and nausea
- blurry vision
- balance problems
- bladder control problems
- thinking and memory problems

> The name hydrocephalus comes from the Greek: *hydro* = water, and *kephale* = head, so it literally means 'water head'.

Leptomeninges

The **leptomeninges** are the two innermost membranes that cover the brain and the spinal cord. They can be affected by neurosarcoidosis, giving rise to meningitis.

Aseptic meningitis

Aseptic means that this form of meningitis is not caused by any infectious agent (like bacteria or viruses), but is caused by the neurosarcoidosis itself.

There are two types of aseptic meningitis seen in neurosarcoidosis:

Acute meningitis is a sudden onset of meningitis, while **chronic meningitis** develops slowly over a few weeks or months. Symptoms of meningitis include a high fever, severe headache, and a stiff neck (so you can't put your chin down to your chest), followed by vomiting and drowsiness, and possible light sensitivity.

Spinal cord

Myelopathy

Myelopathy is a general term for disease of the spinal cord. It is very rare, occurring in less than 1% of neurosarcoidosis patients[6]. It is hard to distinguish between cancerous tumours of the spine and neurosarcoid granulomas, so an accurate diagnosis can be very difficult.

Myelopathy can cause quite severe symptoms, depending on which part of the spinal cord is affected. Symptoms can include leg stiffness, loss of balance, muscle weakness, and bladder problems[5].

Peripheral nerves

The peripheral nervous system is made up of all the nerves that are outside of the brain and spinal cord. It runs through everywhere in your body, and connects your whole body to the central nervous system. Most of the cranial nerves, apart from the optic nerves, are part of the peripheral nervous system.

Cranial neuropathy

This refers to damage to the nerves in the skull (**cranium**), and is the most common manifestation of neurosarcoidosis.

Of these, facial nerve **palsy** (paralysis) is the most common[6]. It is seen in 25–50% of neurosarc patients[28]. It is usually **unilateral** (affecting one side), but can also be bilateral. Facial palsy is usually a short-term complication, and most patients recover from a facial palsy completely. Sometimes it is known as Bell's Palsy.

Trigeminal neuralgia is often seen too — irritation of the fifth cranial nerve. This can cause episodes of sudden, shock-like burning pain on the face, or chronic pain on the face.

Optic neuritis is another common cranial neuropathy, occurring in up to 38% of neurosarc cases. Optic nerve damage results in blurred vision, partial vision loss, or other visual field defects. The loss of vision usually develops over a few hours or a few days.

Around 20% of neurosarc patients have uveitis[7]. This is, broadly speaking, inflammation of the uvea, which is the coloured part of the eye (and can include the iris and retina).

Depending on the exact nerve affected, **cranial neuropathy** can also lead to things like:

- neurological hearing loss
- sense of smell and taste loss or impairment
- facial tics or spasms
- difficulty speaking
- difficulty swallowing
- double vision
- drooping eyelids
- vertigo
- pain
- tingling
- numbness

Peripheral neuropathy

Peripheral neuropathy is a general term meaning 'damage to the peripheral nerves'. This damage can be caused by an injury, or a disease, or for other reasons. In this instance, peripheral neuropathy is caused by the action of neurosarcoidosis.

Peripheral neuropathy may be unilateral or bilateral, affect the large nerves, or the smallest nerves (**small fibre neuropathy**). It may affect only one nerve, or many. It can sometimes affect the **autonomic** nerves — the nerves that control non-voluntary muscles, like the heart, bladder and intestines.

Peripheral neuropathy from neurosarcoidosis generally affects many nerves, not just one. Defects in the function of one or more of the senses (**sensory deficit**) are more common than problems with muscle movement. Chronic pain is one of the most commonly reported symptoms in neurosarc patients. This might be caused by small fibre neuropathy, which causes pain, numbness, burning sensations, and vibrating or shock-like feelings[1].

Because our peripheral nerves do so many things, damage to these nerves can result in a lot of different symptoms. Some examples are:

- muscle weakness
- muscle loss
- bone degeneration
- changes in skin, hair and nails
- numbness
- difficulty walking
- poor balance
- reduced or lost reflexes
- phantom sensations (e.g. of wearing gloves, when you're not)
- reduced sense of touch
- reduced ability to feel pain
- reduced ability to sense temperature
- reduced sense of smell and taste
- phantom smells

- heightened sensitivity, so normal touch becomes painful (eg sheets on legs)
- dry eyes and/or mouth
- tiredness
- tingling
- pain
- itching
- crawling sensations
- pins and needles
- muscle twitching
- cramps
- tremor

Symptoms of autonomic peripheral neuropathy can include:

- heat intolerance from an inability to sweat normally
- loss of bladder control
- inability to manage blood pressure, which can lead to dizziness or fainting (postural or orthostatic hypotension)
- digestive upsets, diarrhoea, constipation, incontinence
- difficulty eating or swallowing
- sexual dysfunction, leading to things like erectile dysfunction, impotence, and decrease in vaginal lubrication

Myopathy

Myopathy is a general term for 'disease of muscle tissue'. Sometimes sarcoidosis nodules form within muscle tissue.

Myopathy does develop in 50–80% of neurosarc patients, but in almost all cases it doesn't cause muscle problems. Less than 3% of patients have actual symptoms of muscle disease from sarcoidosis, so it's very unusual for it to cause symptoms. 'Active' myopathy from NS tends to be chronic, which can cause slowly worsening muscle weakness and **atrophy** of some muscles[7].

Functional neurological symptoms

It's common to have a bunch of niggling neurological symptoms that come and go. Maybe one arm gets painful to touch for a day. Or you get a hand tremor. Or a foot starts buzzing, twitching, or going numb. Or you get dizzy all of a sudden. Or a host of other things. When you have a neurological disease like neurosarcoidosis, this is naturally worrying. Is this some new manifestation of the disease?

However, your doctors may well gloss over these symptoms, leaving you feeling unheard and frustrated. There is a reason for this apparently blasé attitude — they're not ignoring you or your new symptoms, and these symptoms *are* real — but your doctors may suspect that these are not symptoms that mean your disease is worsening, or that you have new sarc **lesions**. These sorts of symptoms are often what's known as functional neurological symptoms.

Functional symptoms tend to flare up for a little while, but then settle down quickly. They can be likened to a 'software' problem with the nervous system — while the disease activity of neurosarc is more of a 'hardware' problem.

The cause of functional symptoms isn't clear in many cases. They might be the result of old healed damage to the nerve sheaths from sarcoidosis. These scarred areas might get inflamed, or cause the nerve to not work frightfully well for a little while. So they are more likely to be the result of *past* damage, rather than evidence of new disease activity. These symptoms typically flare and settle down fairly quickly, within a day or so.

How can you tell when a new symptom is something to be concerned about?

Serious disease activity in neurosarcoidosis tends to develop and worsen over hours or several days, and *stay bad for days to weeks*. It won't come and go over a few hours or a few days. So if you get a new symptom that follows a pattern of worsening and *staying* bad for days to weeks, that's the time to contact your specialist.

The Functional and Dissociative Neurological Symptoms website by Consultant Neurologist Dr Jon Stone discusses functional neurological symptoms in greater depth: **www.neurosymptoms.org**

General symptoms and signs

Nonspecific symptoms can occur in many chronic autoimmune and inflammatory diseases. They are not specific to neurosarcoidosis (so not of much help when it comes to diagnosis), but they are symptoms you may well have. Some of these may be functional neurological symptoms (see above):

- fatigue
- malaise — general feeling of illness
- headaches (seen in nearly half of NS patients[1])
- dizziness
- brittle hair, hair loss
- slight fever
- onycholysis — painless lifting of the nails from the nail bed
- deformed nails

- rough surface to nails
- decreased reflexes
- positive blood test results (ANA, CRP, ESR) — see Chapter 2

Prognosis

We all want to know what the future holds for us when we get a diagnosis of neurosarcoidosis. It's pretty damn frightening, after all, having a disease that affects our brain and nerves!

Unfortunately, no doctor can tell you exactly what your future with neurosarc will be like. There are many different sorts of neurosarc.

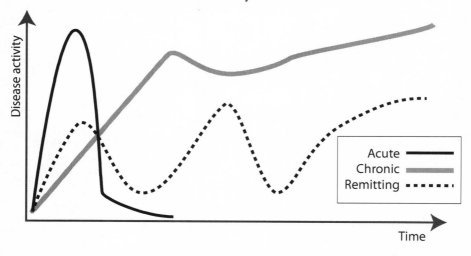

Figure 3 — Patterns of disease in neurosarcoidosis over time
After Pardo[12]

This disease isn't well understood, and everyone has different collections of symptoms and reactions to treatment, and possibly other conditions that complicate matters.

Figure 3 illustrates the different 'disease paths' that neurosarcoidosis can take.

Neurosarcoidosis can present in three general patterns of disease activity over time[12]: acute, chronic, or relapsing-remitting.

With acute NS, patients typically have one single episode of cranial nerve involvement or meningitis, and the disease then goes into remission.

With chronic NS, the disease gradually worsens over time.

With relapsing-remitting NS, the disease has times when it's flared and active, and then times of remission with low disease activity, in a repeating 'on and off' cycle.

Patients may start with 'regular' sarcoidosis, or develop sarcoidosis in other parts of their body later (and often do), so this makes the whole picture of each individual's neurosarcoidosis more complicated.

The research to date reveals the following generalisations, depending on what sorts of neurosarcoidosis symptoms you get.

Those with central nervous system (brain and spinal cord) involvement generally have worse outcomes than those who only have peripheral nervous system involvement. There is a 10% death rate from neurosarcoidosis, twice that from 'general' sarcoidosis[5]. 90% of patients survive.

Progression means the worsening of a disease. This may mean that symptoms you already have become more severe, and/or that you develop new symptoms of the disease.

Figure 4 on the next page shows the relative severity of different neurosarc symptoms. Please keep in mind that these are *general* findings, averaged over many patients, and doesn't mean that *you* in particular are doomed.

The neurosarcoidosis symptoms which are the least cause for concern, and a low risk for progression of the disease are at the bottom of the list. However,

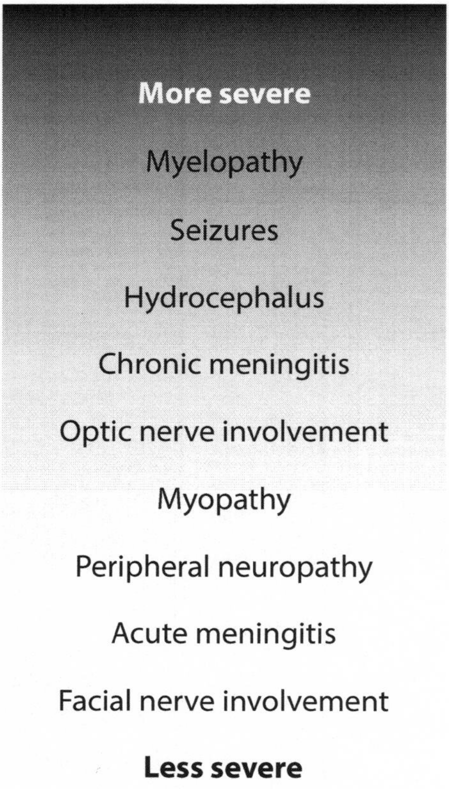

More severe

Myelopathy

Seizures

Hydrocephalus

Chronic meningitis

Optic nerve involvement

Myopathy

Peripheral neuropathy

Acute meningitis

Facial nerve involvement

Less severe

Figure 4 — Relative severity of neurosarcoidosis symptoms

just because a symptom is listed as 'less serious' doesn't necessarily mean that it *won't* progress, it just means that it's less *likely* to progress.

Symptoms listed at the top of Figure 4 are the most cause for concern, and are linked to the most serious progression of the disease. But if you have one of these symptoms, it doesn't mean your neurosarcoidosis *will* progress. It just means that it's more likely that it will[1].

2
Diagnosis

The current state of neurosarcoidosis diagnosis is discussed in this chapter. There is always research being done into neurosarcoidosis, so hopefully in the future there will be new ways of approaching diagnosis, arising from a better understanding of this difficult disease.

Diagnosis of neurosarcoidosis is a complex and difficult task. One clinic reports that the average time it takes to get a diagnosis, after the start of neurological symptoms, is roughly two to four years[13]. Many patients report much longer times.

Early symptoms may be dismissed by doctors — neurological symptoms can be vague and it isn't always clear that they mean anything in particular, in the early stages. It can take a long time to be taken seriously and to get in to see a specialist. Neurological diseases in general are hard to diagnose, and often many years need to go by before symptoms become clear enough to pin down a diagnosis.

Most doctors don't know a lot about neurosarcoidosis, and some can even be dismissive, which only compounds these problems. Often it takes a dramatic worsening of symptoms, some sudden medical crisis that results in hospitalisation, before a patient is really investigated thoroughly for neurological, inflammatory, and autoimmune diseases.

One problem is that early symptoms of NS can be very nonspecific and vague. Mild neurological symptoms and signs can occur in anyone, any time; and *most* of the time they don't signify anything particularly bad (see page 18 about functional neurological symptoms).

There are many other diseases that are more likely to be the cause of neurological symptoms, than neurosarc. They need to be excluded first. One of the biggest dilemmas for specialists is trying to figure out whether an infection is causing your symptoms or not. And even if granulomas are discovered, this doesn't mean you have sarcoidosis. Granulomas can form in many other diseases, so the presence of granulomas doesn't mean they're caused by sarcoidosis[28].

Multiple sclerosis (MS), vasculitis, lupus, tumours, **Lyme disease**, **Behcet's disease**, central nervous system **lymphoma, Wegener's granulomatosis**, tuberculosis, and infections, among others, need to be ruled out. And many of *these* diseases are rare and hard to diagnose too, which only compounds the problems of settling on a diagnosis.

Multiple sclerosis in particular overlaps a great deal with neurosarcoidosis, in terms of test results and symptoms, so it is common to have MS suggested at various points in the process of getting a diagnosis[1].

There are no definitive blood tests or scans to detect neurosarcoidosis; your doctors have to gradually build up a picture of what they think the most *likely* diagnosis is. Diagnosis with neurosarc is usually phrased as 'possible NS', 'probable NS', or 'definite NS'.

If you have sarcoidosis elsewhere in your body that can help with diagnosis, as it's easier to get a biopsy from these areas. It is also suggestive of NS if you already have sarcoidosis elsewhere (although sarcoidosis patients can have neurological symptoms that are *not* caused by neurosarcoidosis[1]). Doctors also don't tend to go barging in taking tissue samples of your brain to see if it's NS (although this is occasionally done), as this is a very invasive procedure.

So, diagnosis is an extremely complicated, lengthy and difficult process, and prone to errors. Your doctors may change their minds along the way. This is a reflection on the difficulty of making a clear diagnosis at all, not poor medical training.

Scans and tests

Radiation

Some of the tests you may have involve exposure to ionising radiation of various types. MRIs and ultrasound scans involve very little radiation exposure. The amount of radiation you're exposed to with an x-ray or CT scan is minimal. Gallium and PET scans have higher levels of exposure.

Every day we are exposed to background radiation from our surroundings, from sources such as the sun, space, and soil, to the rocks under our feet and radon gas — we are even exposed to higher levels during air travel. Radiation exposure is often discussed in terms of 'how many days/months/years of background radiation this is equivalent to'.

A chest x-ray is equivalent to about 10 days of background radiation, and a CT scan of the head is equivalent to 8 months[29]. Both of these scans involve low exposure. A PET scan is equivalent to about 8 years of exposure to background radiation, and a gallium scan is equivalent to about 10 years[30]. So, as you can see, PET and gallium scans involve much higher radiation exposure.

The risk of developing health problem as a result of exposure to radiation from these sorts of scans is low, but your doctors may avoid sending you for gallium or PET scans every year.

Magnetic resonance imaging (MRI)

MRI is the best scanning method used so far to detect neurosarcoidosis lesions. It is very good at looking at the soft structures of the body, and can highlight areas of inflammation. The best results are obtained from MRIs done 'with contrast', which means a special contrast dye (gadolinium) — often called an 'agent' — is injected into you during the scan. This helps to improve the detail of the scans. MRIs use magnetic fields, so you receive no exposure to ionising radiation from them.

An MRI scanner has a long tunnel, roughly 1.5 metres (5') long. The tunnel is narrow — only around 70 cm (28") across. You lie on a long table that very slowly moves you through the scanner. Scans may take up to an hour or longer.

Because of the massive magnetic fields, you must not wear any magnetic metal during an MRI, and the technicians will ensure that you're safe before going in to the scanner. If you have a pacemaker, you probably won't be able to have an MRI. Artificial joints and IUDs do not present a problem. Magnetic fields can not harm or affect you otherwise.

The roof of the MRI tube is quite close to your face, and a lot of people find the enclosed space very challenging to cope with. The tube is lit, and a lot of MRI scanners blow a gentle breeze through the tube, to help you feel less claustrophobic.

During the scan, the machine makes very loud clunking, thumping and clicking sounds (all perfectly normal), so you will be given ear plugs or possibly headphones to listen to music. If you're having a brain MRI, your head may be strapped or clamped into a frame, and foam wedges may also help to hold your head still.

Coping with MRIs

Brain and spinal MRIs can take a long time, up to an hour or more. If you have trouble dealing with being in an enclosed space during an MRI scan, or find the clamps on your head painful (they may feel fine at first, but after a while the constant pressure can hurt), the following tips may help you:

- Ask for a mild **sedative** from your specialist or GP well before the scan, something like diazepam (Valium), and discuss what options are available. Take it half an hour or so before the scan, and make sure the MRI technicians know that you've taken it. You will also need someone to bring you to and from the scan, as you mustn't drive if you've taken a sedative medication.

- Use meditation or mindfulness techniques to calm yourself during the scan. Some facilities can pipe music through to you, using their own non-magnetic headphones.

- Keep your eyes closed during the scan.

- Ask if your head has to be clamped or not. It may be possible to avoid the clamps, and just use foam blocks and wedges to keep your head still during the scan.

- If your head has to be clamped, ask if they can put extra padding under the clamps.

Computed tomography (CT)

A computed tomography (CT) scan uses x-rays and computers to create a very detailed two or three dimensional image. It is sometimes called a CAT scan (computed axial tomography). Unlike other imaging methods, CT scans can show all types of body structures at once — bones, blood vessels, organs, soft tissues. A CT scan involves some exposure to ionising radiation, but not a lot.

Having a CT scan is easy. The scanner has a table to lie on, and a thin ring structure which holds the x-ray source and detectors. The table slowly slides you through the ring during the scanning process. During the scan the machine makes a whooshing and swishing sound, but it's not very loud. There is no long tunnel, so you shouldn't have any problems with claustrophobia.

You may need to have some contrast dye injected before or during the scan, through a **cannula** (a thin tube inserted into a vein). The contrast dye can make you feel flushed for a minute, cause a metallic taste in your mouth, and make you feel like you've wet yourself (rest assured, you haven't). A scan takes anywhere from a few minutes to half an hour, depending on the area to be scanned.

Positron emission tomography (PET)

Positron emission tomography (PET) scans produce a three dimensional image of your body. A PET scan can reveal the extent of disease throughout the body, and helps rule out other possible causes of symptoms.

It is an effective and sensitive scanning method, but an expensive one. A PET scan also involves moderately high exposure to ionising radiation, so it is unlikely your doctors would request this scan frequently for both of these reasons.

A PET scan can take from 20 minutes to an hour. The scanner consists of a table you lie on, and a large detector ring, which you are passed through. The ring is quite narrow, but is not an enclosed space.

A relatively new diagnostic scan is the use of $[^{18}F]$-fluorodeoxyglucose (FDG) PET scans to identify good sites for biopsy of sarcoidosis granulomas, and to reveal the extent and age of granulomas. It can show whether lesions are old or new, which is very useful information.

^{18}F-FDG is a radioactive sugar, which breaks down rapidly. The process involves having an injection of the ^{18}F-FDG solution by IV, after fasting for at least 6 hours. You then rest for about an hour for the solution to be taken up through your body, and have the scan.

Lumbar puncture (spinal tap)

Lumbar puncture is done to sample some of the fluid in your spinal column (cerebrospinal fluid, or CSF). It is a good way to see if there are any abnormalities. It can help in the diagnosis of neurosarcoidosis, multiple sclerosis, infectious meningitis, and some other diseases. The pressure of the CSF is also measured. It can also sometimes be used to inject dyes or anaesthetics into the central nervous system. Keep in mind that 20–33% of neurosarc patients have normal CSF[8] — so it is possible to get negative lumbar puncture results, and still have the disease.

A range of things are looked for in the CSF sample, including:

- antibodies (immunoglobulins) in the fluid. These are detected using electrophoresis gels — they show up as particular stripes (**oligoclonal bands**) on the gels.
- white blood cells levels
- glucose levels
- infectious agents

A lumbar puncture involves having a tiny needle inserted into your spine, and some of the cerebrospinal fluid removed for analysis. The test is often done in your hospital bed, or may be done under CT scan or **fluoroscopy** (use of live x-ray imaging to guide the positioning of the needle). The test usually takes about half an hour.

You lie on your side, curled up, with your back to the doctor. A local anaesthetic is used to numb the area, and great care is made to make sure everything is sterile. The doctor will then insert a very fine needle into the spinal canal, and samples of the CSF are taken.

Lumbar puncture can be uncomfortable or painful, although sometimes it can be practically painless, in the hands of a skilled operator. Regardless of the experience of the doctor, it is possible for the test fail, or need to be repeated, as it is a difficult test to do successfully.

The main possible side effect is a headache after the procedure, which around 30% of patients develop; lying down flat for some hours after the procedure might help to ease the pain of the headache, but won't necessarily stop it.

Tissue biopsy

A tissue sample that has sarcoidosis granulomas in it is the 'gold standard' for a diagnosis of sarcoidosis. The **pathologist** will be able to look at the sample under a microscope and see whether sarcoidosis granulomas are there or not.

However, with neurosarcoidosis it's very hard to get a sample of brain or nerve tissue, and most of the time this isn't done because of the risk to the patient.

If you have evidence of sarcoidosis elsewhere in your body, such as skin lesions, or lung involvement, then a tissue sample may be taken from one of these other areas, to see if sarcoidosis is present elsewhere in your body. If it is, then it makes it more likely that your neurological symptoms are also being caused by sarcoidosis (although not absolutely certain).

How the tissue biopsy is done will depend on what area of the body needs to be sampled. Most biopsies are done using a hollow needle to sample the tissue. Sometimes a CT or ultrasound scanner is used to help guide the position of the needle. Skin biopsies may be done with a scalpel, too. You should be given some local anaesthetic before the procedure, and you may need pain relief afterwards.

X-ray

An x-ray of the lungs may be done to see if there is any evidence of sarcoidosis in the lungs (which is very common, see page 7). An x-ray is a common scan, and involves low exposure to radiation.

During an x-ray you will be asked to stand in front of a plate, or lie on a table. You will need to hold your breath while the x-ray is taken, which only takes a few seconds. It is a quick and easy scan.

Gallium scan

A gallium scan can show whether lesions are new or old, which is very helpful information for doctors. It pinpoints areas where there is rapid cell division in the body, which can indicate infection, injury, inflammation, or cancer.

It does involve moderately high exposure to radiation; the gallium gives off gamma rays. It is not great for detecting neurosarcoidosis, but is very useful in detecting other sarcoidosis granulomas elsewhere in the body.

A small dose of radioactive gallium is injected into you several hours or even days before the scan. When it's time to come back for your scan, you lie still on the scanner bed. The scanner camera then moves slowly above the bed to complete the scan. There are no enclosed spaces, although the scanner plate can come very close to your face. If this is a problem for you, simply close your eyes for the time the scanner plate is over your face. The scan may take up to an hour or so.

Nerve conduction study

This test is carried out by a neurologist, or within a hospital, and tests how well your nerves are working. It can be easily done, and is non-invasive.

You need to avoid putting on any skin cream on before a nerve conduction test. Surface electrodes are stuck onto your skin in particular places on your limbs, and small electric currents are pulsed through the electrodes to activate the nerves. The reaction of your nerves to the stimuli is recorded through several other electrodes on your skin.

The test can be uncomfortable or even quite painful at times, from the mild electric shocks. But there are usually no needles involved, and it is also quite a short test, so it will be over with quickly.

The main failing of this test is that it only tests the functioning of large nerves, and doesn't test small nerve fibres. These small nerves are typically the ones damaged in small fibre **neuropathy,** which can be present in neurosarcoidosis[5]. So it is possible to have a normal nerve conduction study, but still have neuropathy.

Less common tests

There are a wide range of possible additional tests that can be done. Below are a few of these, but they are not the only ones.

Bronchoalveolar lavage (BAL)

If you have sarcoidosis in the lungs, a BAL test can be useful. Lavage means 'washing'. So the lungs are being 'washed' (in just a tiny area), in effect. The goal is to obtain a sample of lung cells.

This is done by passing a long thin instrument (**bronchoscope**) through the nose or mouth into the lungs (you will be sedated), and a little fluid is squirted into a small area of the lungs. This fluid, and the cells that have washed away, are then collected up, and analysed.

Cerebral angiogram

This exam investigates how the blood flows inside the brain. It is done under local anaesthetic and a sedative. A very thin flexible catheter (tube) is passed from your groin up through the arteries to your neck. Then a special contrast dye is injected into the catheter, and x-ray scans are used to track how the blood moves through the brain.

Lymph node biopsy

Lymph nodes are small organs of the immune system. They are full of white blood cells and act as traps for antigens. You have about 500–600 lymph nodes scattered through your body.

A biopsy of a lymph node is a minor surgical procedure that usually removes a whole lymph node, or possibly a tissue sample from one. Looking at these samples can help to diagnose immune and inflammatory diseases.

Q-SART

The Q-SART test stands for the Quantitative Sudomotor Axon Reflex Test (Q-SART is simpler, isn't it!). This test looks at small fibre peripheral nerve function (which isn't tested by a nerve conduction study). It helps to assess autonomic nervous system disorders and peripheral neuropathies.

This is a non-invasive test. It works by looking at the nerves that control sweating. Electrodes filled with **acetylcholine** are placed on particular places on your body (leg and wrist), and then an electric current is passed through them, and your sweat responses are measured. The test takes about 45 minutes, and you may feel some mild burning sensation where the electrodes are.

Visual evoked potential (VER)

This is a test that can help to diagnose problems with the optic nerves. It involves having electrodes placed on your scalp, and then watching checkerboard patterns flash on a screen for several minutes, one eye at a time. The electrical signals from your brain produced as a result of watching these patterns are recorded and analysed. It is a test often used in diagnosing multiple sclerosis.

Blood tests

Here is an explanation of the more common blood tests you will see on your doctor's blood test request forms.

FBC : Full Blood Count

Also called: Full Blood Examination (FBE), Full Blood Picture (FBP), Complete Blood Count (CBC), Complete Blood Examination (CBE), and Complete Blood Picture (CBP).

This is one of the most common blood tests. It simply gives a breakdown of the kinds and amounts of the different cells in your blood. Red blood cells, white blood cells, and **platelets** are assessed, as well as your level of **haemoglobin** (the protein that carries oxygen in your red blood cells).

There are many reasons for having a FBC test, and your doctor may well include it on every blood test you have. It can help see whether you have an infection, help monitor how you're coping on a particular drug, reveal if you're **anaemic**, and many other things.

ESR : Erythrocyte Sedimentation Rate

This is the rate at which your red blood cells (**erythrocytes**) settle at the bottom a test tube over an hour. If the rate they collect is faster than usual, it can indicate there is some inflammation going on.

ESR is a non-specific test, which means it doesn't tell you much more than the fact there is inflammation. A non-specific test cannot tell you which disease is present.

CRP : C-Reactive Protein

C-reactive protein is a protein found in the blood. Its role is to bind to damaged, dead or dying cells, starting the immune response. If there is inflammation in your body, CRP levels are elevated. It is a more sensitive test for inflammation than ESR, but is still pretty non-specific. Having an elevated CRP indicates you have inflammation, but not anything more than that.

ANA : Anti-Nuclear Antibodies

Anti-nuclear antibodies are antibodies that act against the body's own proteins, and bind to the nucleus of cells.

Normally white blood cells should not start an immune response against cells from our own body. In autoimmune diseases, this process fails, and antibodies are produced against your own cells. Your immune system is seeing these cells as antigens, although they are not. So, if an autoimmune disease is present, there will *probably* be higher levels of ANAs in your blood. ANA may also be high in inflammatory diseases, like neurosarcoidosis.

The ANA blood test is done by diluting your blood sample until there is no sign of the ANAs left in the sample. Each dilution doubles the number. The results are given as a ratio, such as 1:80, 1:160, 1:320, and 1:1,280. Results over 1:160 are generally viewed as a positive result.

ANA is a non-specific test, as many autoimmune and inflammatory diseases will give a positive reading — and some healthy people have elevated ANA results for no obvious reason.

This means that if you have a positive ANA, you *might* have an autoimmune or inflammatory disease. The test can't pinpoint which one, and it's possible you might not have anything wrong at all! Not everyone who has an autoimmune or inflammatory disease will have a positive ANA, either. But it is still a useful test to do, especially when combined with other tests such as ACE, ESR and CRP. Just don't pay *too* much attention to the number.

ACE : Angiotensin Converting Enzyme

ACE is a blood test that detects granuloma-producing diseases, and is mainly used to help in the diagnosis of sarcoidosis. It can be elevated in other granuloma-producing diseases too, such as leprosy, **asbestosis**, and tuberculosis.

Angiotensin converting enzyme (ACE) is an enzyme made by blood vessel cells that help regulate blood pressure — it causes blood vessels to contract. The name ACE maybe familiar to you — if you have high blood pressure, you may be on ACE inhibitor medication.

However, ACE is also often secreted by cells in the outside margins of granulomas. So if a granuloma-causing disease is active, ACE levels can be elevated, because the granulomas are making more ACE than you'd normally have.

About 50–80% of patients with active sarcoidosis will have higher levels of ACE. However, 20–50% of the time there is no sign of high ACE levels, despite sarcoidosis being present. ACE levels are also *less* likely to be high in patients with chronic sarcoidosis (such as neurosarcoidosis), so ACE isn't that useful in the diagnosis or tracking of neurosarc, unfortunately.

Lower ACE readings mean that your condition is improving, and higher ACE levels mean that the disease is becoming more active, or that treatment isn't working as effectively. However, tracking neurosarcoidosis with ACE levels is only occasionally useful.

Other blood tests

Elevated vitamin D often leads to an increase in serum levels of calcium. Vitamin D levels do give valuable information on the number of granulomas present. Calcium levels are related to vitamin D levels.

There is an excellent website that can explain your other blood tests to you, Lab Tests Online. The site is available for many different countries (as different countries sometimes call the same tests different names). Just select your country on this website: **labtestsonline.org**

3
Treatment

The current state of treatment for neurosarcoidosis is discussed in this chapter. Hopefully in the future there will be new treatments for this horrid disease.

Some forms of 'general' sarcoidosis that don't affect the nervous system do not require any treatment, but neurosarcoidosis almost always does need treatment.

Neurosarcoidosis is mostly treated with immune suppressant medications. All medical studies of neurosarcoidosis patients over many years have demonstrated their effectiveness.

Corticosteroids are one of the cornerstones of treatment, but their difficult side effects limit their use. Therefore, other drugs with similar immunosuppression effects will often be used. These immune suppressant medications are generally tolerated a lot better than steroids, with many fewer side effects, and most patients can get good control and high rates of improvement in their symptoms[8]. Sometimes patients are prescribed steroids and immune suppressants at the same time.

As you read this section, it's worth keeping the words of Dr Mark Crislip in mind: "Any therapy worth its salt is going to have the potential to hurt you. Sorry. Welcome to medicine. There are always too many overlaps of the sites of drug action to think they will only work on one problem with no side effects ... The more dangerous a drug, the more likely it is to be of benefit." [35]

For all of the drugs discussed below, please follow *your* doctor's advice on the dose *you* need, what side effects to look out for, and read the medication information that comes with each drug you're on. Your pharmacist is also a good source of information and advice.

Corticosteroids

Also called: steroids, cortisone, prednisolone, prednisone, often shortened to 'pred'. Or 'that @!*$ drug'.

Corticosteroids are a group of hormones that your body produces naturally. They are made in the **adrenal cortices**, which are part of the adrenal glands on top of your kidneys. These hormones are involved in the stress response, immune system, dealing with inflammation, **metabolism** of carbohydrates, the breakdown of proteins, blood **electrolyte** levels, and behaviour.

Corticosteroids are the usual first treatment for neurosarc. Steroids are very effective at controlling NS, and even reversing its effects. However, the side effects of this medication are often highly unpleasant and can even be permanently damaging.

Patients with less serious symptoms, who have a low risk of the disease progressing, usually respond well to short courses of corticosteroids. Patients with more severe symptoms often need high doses and/or long courses of these steroids[3].

Some people will need very high doses initially to repair damage from neurosarc, either orally or intravenously. For oral doses, this is typically on a tapering dose, so you might start on, say, 60 mg for a month, and then drop down to 50 mg for the next month, and keep reducing the dose this way. At lower doses, steroid doses are typically reduced at a much slower rate, such as 1 mg/week.

Tapering has to be done slowly. When you take corticosteroids, you're replacing the corticosteroids that your body naturally makes. Your body stops making it, because there's suddenly this nice easy external source of the hormones — one less thing to do!

So if you stop your prednisolone suddenly, your body isn't ready and can't suddenly start making the hormones again. This is extremely dangerous; you can go into **adrenal crisis**, which makes you extremely ill and can be fatal. So it's *vital* to taper your dose of prednisolone slowly, as frustrating as this can be … your body has to slowly realise that it needs to produce the corticosteroids again by itself, and start doing it. Follow your doctor's advice on tapering to the letter.

High steroid doses can also be given for short 'pulse' doses of a few days, or over a few weeks, to settle flares of the disease. In these cases either a taper isn't required, or is done quickly over a week or two. This is safe for very short courses of the steroids.

Side effects

Corticosteroids have a vast list of possible side effects, which is why your doctors are likely to try to get you on a reduced dose, or off them altogether, and onto 'steroid-sparing' medication (more on this below). Your doctor may prescribe calcium and/or potassium supplements while you are on corticosteroids.

Weight gain

This is the biggie, pardon the bad joke. Weight gain while taking corticosteroids is almost inevitable. Even if by some miracle you don't gain weight, *where* your body stores fat will change. The classic 'Cushingoid' appearance is a moon face, fat neck, and more weight on your body and neck, with less weight on the arms and legs. A 'camel hump' at the back of the neck often develops too.

Your appetite typically increases while taking pred. It really doesn't help matters when you feel like eating *everything* in the fridge. With whipped cream on top. Chapter 5 contains some ideas about managing your weight while on prednisolone.

Other side effects

Weight-gain isn't the only side effect of corticosteroids. This is a list of the more common ones:

- muscle cramps or pain
- muscle weakness
- stretch-marks
- thin and fragile skin
- easy bruising
- poor healing of wounds
- susceptibility to infections
- menstrual abnormalities
- impotence
- acne
- thinning hair on head
- increased hair growth on body
- protruding eyeballs
- nausea
- reflux / heartburn
- peptic ulcers
- thrush
- fatty liver
- high blood pressure
- insomnia
- changes in mood
- irritability, anger

Some of the more serious and long-term complications include:

- steroid-induced diabetes (this generally stops when you stop the medication)

- osteoporosis — taking a calcium supplement can help avoid this
- **cataracts**
- **glaucoma**
- loss of blood supply to the ends of bones, leading to arthritic problems
- suppression of growth in children

Corticosteroids can have a few positive side effects, apart from suppressing neurosarcoidosis and repairing its damage, so let's leave this section on a slightly higher note:

- lovely soft skin
- increased energy

It is important to remember that this medication, while it does have a raft of awful side effects, can help your health a great deal. It is very hard to accept the side effects and especially the changes in your face and body, and it can all be desperately depressing.

Addressing the serious damage from neurosarcoidosis needs to come before the relatively less serious side effects from the steroids. The bottom line is that steroids are very effective for neurosarcoidosis.

I recommend the book *Coping with Prednisone* by sisters Dr Julie Ingelfinger and Eugenia Zuckerman. It has a lot of information about living with corticosteroids, and managing their side effects.

Other immune suppressants

Your specialist is likely to either start you on one of these immune suppressants at the same time as corticosteroids, or gradually wean you off the steroids and onto one of these.

These medications are called '**steroid-sparing agents**'. This means that they allow you to get the same, or better, effect from the steroids you're on, at a much lower dose of the corticosteroids. This helps to reduce the side effects from the steroids. And you may be able to get completely off steroids, and just use these medications to control your neurosarc.

As your immune system is being suppressed, it's best to avoid being around people who are sick or have infections (this holds for if you're on corticosteroids, too). You should especially avoid being around people with more serious infectious diseases like shingles, even if you have been immunised for chicken pox in the past, for instance.

You also need to be careful about having 'live' vaccines while on these medications — this includes measles, rubella, mumps, yellow fever, and nasal flu vaccines. However, the injected flu vaccine is perfectly safe to have, and worth getting. Check with your doctor if you have any concerns about vaccinations.

All of these medications can harm an unborn baby, so must not be taken if you are pregnant.

Your doctor will probably order regular blood tests while you're on one of these medications, to check how well you're tolerating it.

You can access more in-depth information about all these medications, and their side effects, at the Drugs.com website, **www.drugs.com** (amongst other websites).

Azathioprine

Brand names: Imuran, Azasan, Azamun, Imurel

Azathioprine reduces the action of your immune system. It is used for people with transplanted organs, to stop rejection, and it is used for people with various autoimmune and inflammatory diseases, most notably rheumatoid arthritis — and neurosarcoidosis!

It can affect your fertility, whether you're a man or a woman. It can also increase your risk for developing certain cancers.

Taking azathioprine with food can help reduce nausea from the medication.

Side effects

Common mild side effects of azathioprine are:

- mild upset stomach
- nausea
- diarrhoea
- loss of appetite
- hair loss
- skin rash

If you develop more severe symptoms, such as fever, **jaundice**, vomiting, or painful urination, seek medical help.

Methotrexate

Brand names: Rheumatrex, Trexall

Methotrexate was originally developed to treat cancer, but it is also very effective against a lot of autoimmune and inflammatory diseases when taken at lower doses. It is generally well-tolerated. It makes you more susceptible to infections and reduces the ability of your blood to clot. Avoid drinking alcohol while taking methotrexate.

Methotrexate is usually taken once a week, not every day. You need to take **folic acid** on the other days of the week (but not on the day you take your dose), as methotrexate interferes with the normal production of folic acid in your body.

Side effects

The most commonly reported side effects from methotrexate are:

- mouth ulcers
- blurry vision
- headaches
- dizziness
- fatigue
- vomiting
- upset stomach

If you develop more severe symptoms, such as fever, shortness of breath, dry cough, blood in urine or stools, swelling, or seizures, seek medical help.

Mycophenolate mofetil

Brand names: CellCept, Myfortic

Mycophenolate mofetil reduces the action of the immune system, so it is used for people with transplanted organs, and for people with autoimmune and inflammatory diseases.

Mycophenolate can make birth control pills less effective, so use an additional form of birth control while taking this medication, if you normally take the pill.

It is best taken on an empty stomach, at least one hour before or two hours after food. Avoid taking **antacids** like Mylanta with mycophenolate, as they can affect the absorption of the drug — get your doctor's advice on a good antacid to use, if you need one.

This medication raises your risk of developing cancer, especially skin cancer. Avoid exposure to sunlight, and definitely avoid tanning beds. Wear protective clothing and a hat, and use a SPF 30 (or higher) sunscreen when outdoors.

Try not to stress about it too much, though. The risk of cancer is still relatively low, with lymphoma appearing in less than 1% of patients, and non-melanoma skin carcinoma in 2-4% of patients taking mycophenolate mofetil[18]. Do remember that 20% of Americans and more than *half* of Australians[19] will develop some form of skin cancer in their lifetime, regardless of whether they take immune suppressants or not.

Side effects

Some of the common mild side effects from mycophenolate include:

- nausea, vomiting
- stomach pain
- diarrhoea and/or constipation
- headache
- mild weakness
- swelling of hands or feet
- numbness
- tingling sensations
- anxiety
- insomnia

If you develop more severe symptoms, such as fever, trouble breathing, vomiting, painful urination, or bloody stools, seek medical help.

Less frequently used medications

For more difficult cases of neurosarcoidosis that don't respond well to oral medications, patients can be given intravenous (IV) medication.

Pulse methylprenisolone (IV)

Brand names: Medrol, Solu Medrol

This is a hit of prednisolone delivered by IV. A pulse dose usually means one **infusion** of the drug, once a week, over a period of some weeks or months. It can also be given as short pulse over a few consecutive days, to treat severe symptoms.

Cyclophosphamide

Brand names: Cytoxan, Endocan, Leukeran, Neosar, Procytox, Revimmune

This medication is a 'pro-drug' – when taken it is inactive, and is converted into the active form of the drug in the liver. It is used to treat cancers and some autoimmune diseases. It can be used to treat sarcoidosis if it has reached a severe stage, and other treatments aren't working. Cyclophosphamide can have some quite severe side effects, including kidney damage, so is generally used as a last resort.

Infliximab or adalimumab

Brand names: Remicade, Humira

Infliximab has been quite successful in patients with chronic and severe sarcoidosis that doesn't respond well to corticosteroids[25]. It is usually given as an IV injection once a month, or under the skin (**subcutaneous** injection). Infliximab and adalimumab are both **TNF** inhibitors[26] (see page 5). They are usually used after other options are not successful or not tolerated[23].

Hydroxychloroquine

Brand names: Plaquenil, Dolquine, Quensyl

This medication is an antimalarial drug, and taken orally. Apart from treating malaria, it is also good at reducing inflammation. It is commonly used to treat diseases like lupus and rheumatoid arthritis, and skin lesions and hypercalcaemia in sarcoidosis.

Pentoxifylline

Brand names: Flexital, Trental, Pentox, Pentoxil

Pentoxifylline is a drug that improves peripheral blood flow, and may be used to treat **pulmonary** sarcoidosis.

Complications and home treatments

If you develop complications from neurosarcoidosis such as meningitis, hydrocephalus or seizures, you will need treatment to manage those specific manifestations of your NS. This may mean anti-epileptic medications, or other treatments. Hydrocephalus is often treated with the insertion of a shunt into the brain, to drain the fluid out of the skull and reduce the pressure on the brain. All the possible options for treatment of all possible complications are beyond the scope of this book, but the information is available from your doctors.

Unfortunately, there aren't many things that can be done to help with neuropathic pain or peripheral neuropathies. Some medications like Lyrica may help you, or may not be effective for you. They are worth trying, though. A TENS machine can be helpful for managing painful areas. Ice or heat packs can help to cope with pain, too.

One of the best things you can do to help yourself is to have an exercise program, especially if you're on steroids. It can be the last thing you feel like doing, but it's very important. Discuss this with your doctor, they will be happy to help you develop a manageable program, or point you towards other specialists who can help you.

Exercise doesn't have to involve running or team sports (although you can do them if you feel up to it, of course) — you may like to investigate low-impact activities like walking, seated exercises, swimming, weight lifting, dancing, or cycling. The most important thing is to find something that you enjoy doing, and to do it most days.

Alternative medicine and pseudo–science

There are millions of medical web sites out there, with more appearing every day. Many medical sites provide good, evidence-based medical information and advice. However, there are just as many — if not more — which can lead you astray.

Some well established and trustworthy medical websites include:

- WebMD **www.webmd.com**
- Health Central **www.healthcentral.com**
- Patient.co.uk **www.patient.co.uk**
- myDr **www.mydr.com.au**
- National Institute of Neurological Disorders and Stroke **www.ninds.nih.gov**

With rare incurable diseases that are disabling, poorly understood, and hard to treat, it's no surprise that some people look for answers in less traditional circles. This certainly holds true with neurosarcoidosis.

The Marshall Protocol is a regime for treating sarcoidosis that was developed in Australia by electrical engineer Trevor Marshall. He theorised that bacteria, reacting with vitamin D, shut down the immune system. He believed that this was the root cause of sarcoidosis and a ton of other conditions, from panic attacks and kidney stones to cystic fibrosis. His treatment regime involves avoiding all vitamin D (including sun exposure), and taking long-term antibiotics. Marshall's theories are based on his computer models, not on medical experiments or results.

There is also a multiple sclerosis therapy, developed by Dr David Wheldon, a **neuropathologist** in the UK. He suggests that a bacterium *Chlamydophila pneumoniae* causes multiple sclerosis. Like the Marshall Protocol, his therapy includes long-term use of antibiotics. He suggests that this therapy could be used to treat many other conditions (including sarcoidosis).

Marshall's and Wheldon's theories are not widely accepted by medical researchers or mainstream doctors, as they have not been verified through proper experiments, which is an absolutely basic requirement for any new treatment. The Marshall Protocol, in particular, can be dangerous to patients with more severe disease (as they warn themselves)[16].

A major argument against these treatments is that sarcoidosis and multiple sclerosis are treated effectively with immune suppressants. While these medications aren't a cure, they do at least suppress the diseases and lessen symptoms.

If these diseases were really perpetuated by ongoing infection with bacteria, as Marshall and Wheldon propose, treatment with immune suppressants would make these diseases flare and much *more* severe — which clearly isn't the case. The fact that these diseases *do* respond to immune suppression, and *don't* flare up and get much worse when on immune suppressants, indicates that they are not caused by infectious agents like bacteria.

Check list

Before you spend your hard earned cash on that magnetic mattress or expensive water, follow these guidelines for spotting "quacky" information.

1. The site or publication uses anecdotes, testimonials, or celebrity endorsements to promote its products. Remember the maxim *"The plural of anecdote is not data."* Just because there are a lot of stories, doesn't mean it's proof. A product that relies heavily on patient stories and testimonials is probably unsupported by experimental evidence.

2. They warn you not to trust your doctor, and claim that "the authorities" are suppressing their information. Any "What *they* don't want you to know" sort of line is always a red flag.

3. A product or treatment that is based on ancient wisdom is always suspect — it's a sure thing that it's pseudo-science. The nature of good science and medicine is that new theories are constantly being put to the test, and improved and changed as our understanding of any subject grows. Medical treatments and understanding is always being improved. Centuries-old knowledge (apart from well-established things such as heat and cold helping to ease pain), that hasn't changed in all that time, isn't really something to be proud of!

4. If a treatment or product is first announced through mass media, rather than peer reviewed medical or scientific journals, it's another warning sign. Good medicine is published in science or medical journals first of all, reviewed, discussed, and repeated by other researchers, and then *eventually,* after *years,* becomes a tested treatment, medication, or product for patients.

5. Any claim based on existence of energy fields or life force energy is suspect. No research — and there has been plenty — has *ever* revealed the existence of such forces. Medical treatments or healing treatments based around these sorts of energy fields, like reiki and therapeutic touch, are bogus.

6. Does the claim sound too good to be true? It usually is. Is the deal too good to be true? It usually is. Does it claim to treat a vast range of different conditions? Another warning sign.

7. Does the doctor have legitimate credentials? Check whether their Alma Mater actually exists, or their degrees have been obtained through recognised accreditation institutions. Unscrupulous people *do* get those free PhDs, and make use of them.

8. "All natural" doesn't mean it's safe or healthy (poisonous toadstools, lead, and salmonella are all natural, after all!). Medications — while they do have side effects — have to go through incredibly rigorous safety testing procedures before they're allowed out in public. The most effective medications have side effects, it's unavoidable.

Natural remedies don't necessarily have such testing, may not have their side effects listed anywhere, and may not even be that "pure", but could be contaminated with other substances. There are many cases of Chinese medicines being adulterated with unlisted medicines and other undisclosed active ingredients, for example, which may interact badly with your prescribed medications.

Alternative therapies can certainly be relaxing, or have placebo effects that may help you feel a bit better for a while. If you are still really keen to try an alternative therapy, run it by your doctor or specialist first, just in case it might interfere with your other sarcoidosis treatment. For instance, ginger supplements can interfere with some blood-thinning medications like warfarin. So it's best to be sure, even if it seems harmless to you.

The PDF brochure *'I've got nothing to lose by trying it: Weighing up claims about cures and treatments for medical conditions'*, from **www.senseaboutscience.org/data/files/resources/136/Ive-got-nothing-to-lose_web.pdf** is excellent, and the Quackcast site **www.quackwatch.org** is essential reading.

4
The emotional impact

When you're living with such a difficult, long-term, and often disabling condition as neurosarcoidosis, it's hardly surprising that it has a psychological impact on your life. This chapter covers some of these impacts, and other 'emotional' topics. There are also some tips for coping when you're still working or studying.

Our own responses

Anger

It's a normal reaction to feel angry about your diagnosis and current situation, and how neurosarcoidosis has stuffed up your life. You may feel angry at yourself, at life, at your body, at your doctors, at others who aren't sick.

Depression and anxiety

An increase in anxiety and depression are normal early responses to your diagnosis, and worsening condition. It takes time to adjust. Shock and denial are also common responses.

It's common to go through cycles of acceptance of your condition, and then back into despair. If you find that you're not coming out of these periods of sadness, but are spiralling downwards into deeper depression, losing interest in life and the things you normally enjoy, and having sleep disturbances (especially trouble getting to sleep, and early morning waking), it is a good idea to see your GP.

Common triggers of anxiety attacks are: waiting for test results, the diagnosis of a severely debilitating condition, the shock it produces, having to have unpleasant medical procedures, the side effects of treatment, changes in lifestyle, reduced independence, increase in medical appointments, increased need for help from other people, and increased reliance on therapy and medication.

Fear

Fear is one of the most prevalent and common reactions to diagnosis with neurosarcoidosis. It is frightening to be looking at the rest of your life with these problems and possible disability ahead of you, from a rare and relatively poorly understood disease. There is no clear cut prognosis, so you have no way of knowing what symptoms you might develop, how the disease might progress in your body (if it does progress), or what sorts of procedures and medications you might have to go through.

Grief

It's normal to feel grief at the loss of normal functioning, increase in pain and disability, and acknowledgement that there is something seriously wrong with your body. As with depression, the process of grief can be cyclical when you're dealing with long-term disability — you may go through it repeatedly. If some aspect of your health suddenly gets worse, the whole grief cycle can start again.

Responses from others

We'd all love to have wonderfully supportive family and friends, who are well-informed, who remember everything you tell them, and are there with tea and sympathy when you need it. You might be lucky, and be in this situation!

However, the reality can be quite different. People forget what you've told them, are unsupportive, mightn't have the emotional or physical energy or inclination to try to understand your situation (unintentionally), or may even be downright rude and callous at times.

If you have some friends or family who really don't 'get it', and either belittle your fears and experiences, or want to keep on talking about it when it's clearly distressing you, you may need to get a bit of distance from them now and then.

Either try to explain clearly and with non-confrontational language ('I' statements such as 'I feel upset when you do X' are better than 'You' ones such as 'You never understand!'), or try to arrange your life so you don't need to interact with them quite as much, if at all possible. It is perfectly okay — in fact, it's healthy — to set boundaries about the behaviour that you will tolerate from others, and what you won't. If you search in books or online for 'setting interpersonal boundaries', you will find a wealth of help and information.

If these people really are unavoidable, then try your best to either explain the cause of your distress, set limits with consequences with them ('If you keep doing X, then Y will happen'), or build up a psychological barrier, and try not to let their words and actions intrude. Easier said than done, I know, but when it comes down to it, they don't have a clue what they're talking about with regard to your health and neurosarcoidosis, and you can safely ignore them.

If you *do* find people around you who are supportive, understanding, and compassionate — hang onto them, and treat them well! You can find supportive and understanding communities online, too.

Chronic illness

Acute illness is a sudden and possibly severe illness — developing a bout of the flu, for example. On the other hand, *chronic illness* is an illness that never ends, or fades but keeps coming back. It's a constant presence in your life. Neurosarcoidosis is a chronic illness.

When illness is constant, it affects everything in your life. You often have to deal with chronic pain, serious levels of fatigue, debilitating symptoms, and permanent effects of the disease. You can't do the things you used to be able to do. Your temper suffers, and this can impact on your relationships too.

It's hard when you have to constantly decline invitations, and it's easy to start to feel resentful and apologetic. Don't feel that you constantly need to offer reasons or excuses for why you can't do something. A simple 'I can't do that', or 'Thank you for asking me, but I can't do that at the moment' will suffice.

You may find yourself on the receiving end of some very odd reactions from acquaintances and others, too. Unfortunately, people often have some rather unhelpful responses to illness and disability. Especially when the problem is internal and invisible, and you *seem* to look normal on the surface, people can be surprisingly callous and unsympathetic.

The underlying — and generally unconscious — thoughts they may be having run along the lines of: "Is this person *really* sick, or making it up? I can't *see* anything wrong with them. Are they faking it and trying to trick me? They look fine to me!"

I'm sure you've heard comments like "You look really great!", "You're looking so well today" and others. These sorts of comments — while they might have been intended to make you feel good — generally have the opposite effect, making you feel invalidated, frustrated, and annoyed. Didn't they *listen* to anything you've said before? Don't they *remember* that you're seriously ill?

So, unfortunately, most people will unconsciously doubt the validity of your condition, and go into 'self-protection doubting' mode, rather than offering help or sympathy. Clear visual cues (e.g. using a walking stick or walker, or wearing a 'sarcoidosis awareness' or 'I'm on Pred' t-shirt) can sometimes help a bit. On my car I have a 'Not all disabilities are visible' bumper sticker, for instance (from CafePress).

This general social response to disability and illness can be disheartening. By being constantly sick, you are unconscious] unintentionally presenting a demand on others; you need specia⍳ treatment, consideration, and adaptations, you're different, you need help. People often feel quite inadequate to meet that challenge, and don't know what to say or do.

It's inevitable — when you have a rare medical condition, you can't expect other people to be able to understand what you're going through, or for them to remember that you still have problems a month later. This is just human nature, and something that anyone with *any* chronic condition comes across. You are naturally the expert in your own condition — and let's face it, you wouldn't know about neurosarcoidosis if you didn't *have* neurosarcoidosis!

The 'Spoon Theory', by Christine Miserandino, is a handy way to explain what it's like living with debilitating diseases. You may find it helps you in explaining things to friends and family, when you yet again have to refuse a social invitation because of crushing fatigue and pain. If you search the web for 'Spoon Theory' you will easily find it; it's on the *But You Don't Look Sick* website.
www.butyoudontlooksick.com

You will probably find that the only people who *really* understand your situation are those who also live with chronic illness or pain of some sort, or who are carers for people with chronic illness.

Work and study

Many people with neurosarcoidosis are unable to work or study, unfortunately. Some are able to manage part-time or home-based work or studies, where they can work at their own pace. Fatigue and neuropsychological problems such as memory impairment and foggy thinking can make a lot of work difficult. If you have vision impairment, or trouble with fine motor skills, this adds further challenges.

If you are still able to work or study outside of the home, explaining your situation at your workplace or educational institution can be tricky. You may choose not to inform people about your condition, if you're able to get by at work fairly well. However, you may need a lot of time off work, or special considerations, or modifications to your workload. If this is the case, it is best if at least your immediate supervisor, main teacher, or closest colleagues know about your condition.

Part of this comes down to how well you understand and have accepted your own condition. By reconciling yourself to your situation, and the limitations it poses, you can present a fair and realistic case to your boss as to the restrictions and adaptations you may need in the workplace.

Some things you may want to consider are whether you need any temporary adaptations to your workload or classes, the ergonomics of your workplace, accessibility adaptations (speech recognition software, perhaps?), or your work hours.

Are you able to undertake some of your studies part-time? Using teleconferencing could be a better option for you rather than driving to get to a meeting. Are there more supportive chairs that would make sitting for long periods less painful? Can you do some of your work from home?

It's important to say no to unreasonable demands, if you know that you really can't manage something at the moment. If you're feeling overloaded, look at ways of cutting back. Can you finish work one hour early? Or cut back to four days a week, instead of five? Or are there volunteer commitments you can reduce? Are there committees you can step down from?

If you work in an area which has a human resources department, it is important that you communicate clearly with them as well. You may find it helpful to have some letters from your GP or specialist explaining your situation, and the adaptations that you need at work.

The more self-accepting and at ease you can be about your condition, the more at ease others will be around you. Your colleagues take cues from you about when you need help, and what adjustments to make, and when it's okay to discuss it.

If people don't understand why you're doing less, they may think you're not pulling your weight around the workplace, and get resentful. So it is important to take the time to communicate clearly. This creates more trust within the workplace in general, builds more support for you, and more understanding from them of your situation. But it isn't an easy situation, especially as your neurosarcoidosis isn't about to go away any time soon, and can be unpredictable. And not all workplaces are supportive, unfortunately.

The positive thinking myth

You know what? It's okay to be sad and upset about your situation. It *is* crap, there's no two ways about it. You honestly don't have to be upbeat and cheerful all the time, always putting on a brave face.

There's a myth about the power of positive thinking, which is practically accepted knowledge around the world. However, *no* research — and plenty has been done — clearly demonstrates that thinking positively will change your health outcomes, whether it's neurosarcoidosis, diabetes, or cancer. So don't worry that you're somehow harming your health if you're feeling pessimistic, pissed off, or down about it all.

Mental outlook has no impact on survival rates in cancer, for example. Some studies show a link between happiness and good health, but it did not prove that happiness *causes* the good health — it may simply be that people who are healthy feel happier (not surprisingly)! Other studies show that pessimism or mild depression can lead to longer and healthier lives. And one study showed that in some situations, optimistic people are worse off immunologically. The research certainly isn't clear cut[32].

So rest assured, you aren't harming your recovery or condition if you're having a miserable or grumpy day, or if you're generally a bit of a pessimist.

I recommend reading *Bright-sided* by Barbara Ehrenreich, if you're interested in learning more.

Where a positive attitude *can* help is with how engaged you are in managing your disease, seeing your specialists regularly, following treatment regimes, exercising, and doing your best to live as well as you can.

If you are feeling upbeat, you're more likely to take your medication as prescribed, follow your doctors' advice, look after yourself, and be much easier to live with.

But while these can lead to a better outcome, because you're more involved in and responsible for your own health, simply having a sunny disposition or chanting positive mantras isn't going to ease any aches or pains, or cure your disease.

Coping strategies

It is a good idea to seek professional help if you think things are getting out of hand, if you might be depressed, are having anxiety attacks, or if you're not coping with stress. It is better to start seeking help sooner rather than later, too, as it may take a while to find a practitioner who suits you.

A counsellor of some sort can help you to help deal with these emotions and their impact on your well-being. Look for a psychologist who has experience at helping people who have chronic illness and pain problems.

If you have loss of any basic senses, such as vision, hearing, smell, or taste, I encourage you to seek professional counselling, and look for support groups. There are many groups for people with vision and hearing impairment, but fewer for those with smell and taste problems. The book *Navigating Smell and Taste Disorders* by neurologist Ronald DeVere and Marjorie Calvert is very helpful, as is the UK group Fifth Sense **www.fifthsense.org.uk.**

The overall goal here is a more peaceful acceptance of your condition, and a proactive approach to daily life and treatment, without railing against the inevitable and what you cannot change. There are also suggestions for practical coping strategies in the next chapter, and in Chapter 10.

Four steps to take

1) **Don't deny your symptoms.** Putting them out of your mind won't make them go away. At some level, you need to accept that you *do* have a serious disease, and that you need to live with it, and seek and follow treatment to see an improvement in your quality of life long-term.

I'm sorry to say, you're not likely to wake up one happy day with your neurosarc gone. While it's important to have hope, and research into better treatment is ongoing, the reality is you'll probably have to live with this disease in some form or another for the rest of your life.

2) **Remember that while you are a rare one, you're not alone.** At a guess, roughly 140,000 people in the world have neurosarcoidosis (0.002% of 7 billion). Try to connect with other suffers online — you never know, there may even be someone who lives in the same city as you, who you can meet! There are some support group websites to get you started on the Further Reading list on page 144. Even having one or two neurosarcie friends makes a huge difference.

3) **Try to focus on the bits of you that do work, not the parts that don't.** Maybe you can't run around the playground with your kids, but you *can* play card games with them, and give them lots of hugs. Focus on what you can do, and come up with ways of getting around what you can't do any more. This may take some problem solving, I

know, but there are support systems out there that can help. There are adaptive technologies if you have trouble with vision or hearing. There are aids to help with mobility, and so on.

Look at your situation — some things absolutely can't be changed (wishing and positive thinking aren't going to cure you, sorry to say), so look at what things you just have to accept, and don't waste energy fighting and railing against them.

Look at what things you *can* adapt to, and ways you can do things differently to improve your quality of life.

4) **Try your best to live in the present moment, day by day**. Try not to look *too* far into the unknown and unknowable future, or second-guess what some doctor is going to do or say about your condition, or what some test result means. Don't let your disease define you, or be the complete focus of your life every day. Do things you enjoy, don't put your life on hold. Set yourself challenges. Study something you've always wanted to learn — online if necessary. Do crafts or some other hobby. Volunteer for a group or charity that does work you're passionate about. Spend time with friends and family. You still have a great deal to offer the world, and the people around you, even if it's not what you had in mind before you got sick.

See the further reading on page 143 for websites and books to look into for more information.

5
Proactive strategies

This chapter covers some aspects of living with neurosarcoidosis in brief. There are also more tips and tricks for coping with symptoms in Part II, within patients' stories. There are many good references out there about living with disabilities and autoimmune disease in general, some of which I've listed in the further reading list at the end of the book (see page 143).

Corticosteroids and weight gain

Corticosteroids generally lead to inevitable gain weight, and this is one of their most hated side effects. Part of the problem is they increase appetite a great deal, but it is possible to gain weight even without feeling you're eating a lot more — this can be from fluid retention. It is extremely difficult to manage.

To help limit weight gain while on corticosteroids, if you have an iron will, you might like to try this regime:[15]

- avoid salt
- avoid simple carbohydrates
- keep calories down
- exercise

Reducing salt helps to stem fluid retention while on steroids. This can be very hard to do, but your taste buds *do* adjust after a few weeks of low-salt eating, and food will taste fine again. However, if your sense of smell and taste are affected by the neurosarc, reducing salt will make things taste even *more* bland and tasteless than they already do, so cutting salt may be a difficult thing to attempt!

65

Simple carbohydrates (like sugars, white rice and white flour) are not as good for you, or as filling, as complex carbohydrates. They are high **glycaemic index** (GI) foods, which means they cause your blood sugar to quickly rise to a high level.

Low GI foods give a longer and slower release of sugar into your blood. A low GI diet *may* help you to feel full for longer — which helps you to eat fewer calories over the day, hopefully. Complex carbohydrates, like brown rice, whole grain bread, pasta, and beans, are low GI. There are many websites and cookbooks about low GI eating, which you can investigate. Reducing the amount of carbs you eat overall may help matters too.

An exercise program doesn't need to be difficult or expensive, but it is important for your health while on steroids. Look at the activities you enjoy, and what you're capable of doing within the restrictions of the disease. Even seated exercise can help — there is information on many programs online and in your library.

The intermittent fasting regime, also known as 5:2 (5 days of normal eating and 2 non-consecutive days of restricted calories each week), is showing promising results. Using 5:2, weight loss has been possible for some people while still on steroids. All information about doing intermittent fasting is available freely online. You can read more on Dr Michael Mosley's website: **thefastdiet.co.uk** and the Fast Day website: **www.fastday.com**. Both sites have active and friendly forums.

You may like to use a calorie tracking app or website to track what you eat each day, and try your best to stick within the recommended daily calorie allowance for your height, weight, and activity level most days. The free **myfitnesspal.com** website and app is an excellent place to start, but there are many other options too.

When you get off corticosteroids, if you're able to, it *is* possible to lose the extra weight, although it does take work. Managing what you eat is the key; exercise has been shown *not* to help that much with weight loss, especially in women (although it is extremely good for you, for many *other* reasons)[20–22]. Your weight distribution will hopefully return to normal, and your face will look like you again, although it may take some months after coming off the steroids.

Living with fatigue

Crushing fatigue is a common problem for people with neurosarcoidosis (and many other autoimmune and inflammatory diseases). It's not just 'tired', it's being unable to move because you did half an hour of housework. Or being unable to get out of bed because you went out the night before. Or unable to get out of bed at all.

There are many resources out there about coping with this sort of problem, as it's common to many conditions. There aren't really any magic cures for fatigue of this sort, I'm sorry to say. Simply sleeping more won't fix it — most of the time you feel like a truck's hit you when you wake up anyway.

A few conditions may be contributing to your fatigue levels, so make sure that you're not anaemic, and that your vitamin D isn't too low, for starters. Food intolerances can contribute to fatigue. But when it comes down to it, coping with this level of constant exhaustion generally means learning to live within its limitations, which is difficult.

Pacing yourself is one of the best methods for managing. This means knowing your limits — how much can you do before you *can't* manage? What tips you over the edge?

Make sure you do *less* than this limit as a rule, even on 'good days' when you feel you have more energy. Doing too much on these better days is often the cause of a major crash the next day.

Pushing yourself too hard, when you know you've had it, is another problem, and can even lead to flare ups of your disease. The trick is to have a rest *before* you have to have a rest. Resting means giving *everything* a break — lying down in a quiet room, not surfing the web or reading. You may like to try some mindfulness or meditation practices.

Setting limits

Setting limits means knowing the rules for yourself, and sticking to them as much as you can. It also means letting others know what your rules are!

The sorts of questions to ask yourself are: Are you alert enough to drive a car safely? How far can you drive? How far can you walk? How long can you socialise? How long can you sit at the computer? How much can you read?

Some examples of personal rules:

- don't go out two days in a row
- only go out three days a week at most
- don't go out at nights
- get to bed by 9 pm
- don't accept more than one social engagement a week
- limit social visits to two hours
- limit phone conversations to 10 minutes
- only drive within 20 km (10 miles) of home
- don't drive after dark
- avoid being the organiser or host of family events
- only run two errands, or go to one shop, when out
- have a break after an hour of studying

You will need to set up your own rules that suit you, as you know your situation best of all. You may be able to handle driving a longer distance, but need to get to bed by 8 pm, for instance. There will no doubt be other things you need rules for, such as situations at work or school.

Sticking to these rules yourself is hard enough, but explaining them to other people is even harder! It can be done though. Statements such as these can help:

- I'm sorry, I'd love to come to your party, but I don't go out at nights. Can we get together another time?
- I'm not available that day, would the next day be OK?
- I appreciate you thinking of me, but unfortunately I can't take on extra commitments at the moment.

Remember that you don't have to give an explanation of *why* you're not available — **even if the reason you're not available is that you're resting that day. They don't need to know. It's not up for discussion!**

Some other strategies that can help include:

Having a regular schedule that you know is 'safe'. Stop work at 4 pm. Stop for a proper lunch break at 1 pm. Have a lie down every day at 2 pm. Whatever it is that you need to help you get through the day.

Look at consequences, and know the trade offs — if I go to my cousin's wedding, I know I'll be out of action for a week, but it's worth it, I really don't want to miss this important family event. If I go out late night shopping, I'll be wrecked all weekend, it's probably not worth it. I buy what I need online instead.

Some practical tips for coping with fatigue

- Investigate the minimalism movement, and simplify your life; declutter your belongings, own less, do less. This makes housework easier, if nothing else, as there's less stuff to make a mess with.
- Use an answering machine or message service if you're too tired to take a call. Turn your mobile phone and/or land line off now and then.
- Wash dishes and cook sitting down, rather than standing, if possible.

- Use disability aids where they offer some help to you — tools in the kitchen, long-handled grabbers so you don't have to bend down, long-handled gardening tools, walkers to help when out at the shops, and so on.

- Develop a short list of recipes that are healthy, inexpensive, easy, fast, and you like. Write a standard shopping list that covers these dishes, and just shop for those things. Make double batches and freeze meals.

- Shop for groceries online and have them delivered. Many supermarkets offer this service, and there are specialist 'online only' farmer's market type delivery services.

- Use appliances to make things easier in the kitchen, like a food processor, instead of chopping ingredients by hand.

- If you can afford it, get paid help with the housework and/or gardening, especially with the heavier chores such as vacuuming, washing floors and mowing.

- Avoid ironing — choose clothes that don't need ironing. Hang shirts up immediately after drying, so they don't get creased in the first place.

- Shop for household items, birthday and Christmas gifts online, rather than going to the shops. Or make gifts by hand, if you're good at crafts (you can buy a lot of craft supplies online too).

Work and study

The biggest issues for people with neurosarc who are still working and studying seem to be:

- being out for one day can put you in bed the next day
- working too slowly
- lack of understanding from co-workers, teachers and bosses
- long times needed to learn new things
- inability to handle frequent tight deadlines

- symptoms such as migraines and optic neuritis affecting ability to work
- mental confusion and memory issues — forgetting dates and details, unable to explain things.

Adaptations:

These ideas are possible adaptations that you might be able to set in place:

- flexible working hours, avoiding rush deadlines and high pressure projects
- change your work schedule, to work fewer days in a week, or in a job sharing arrangement
- furniture adaptations: highbacked chairs, foot stools and the like
- voice recognition software, if you have vision problems
- change from an active job to an office job
- get up and move regularly
- do volunteer work instead of a paid job

In the USA, you can file a letter under Americans with Disabilities Act, advising your employer that you have this disease, and describing your issues. This Act prohibits discrimination and guarantees that people with disabilities have the same opportunities as everyone else.

Don't worry too much about drug testing. These tests by employers are looking for non-prescription drug use. If your prescription is on file at a pharmacy, you will pass any drug-testing requirements.

There are a few websites listed at the end of the book (page 145) about disability rights in various countries, and your rights as a worker. If your country isn't listed, do a web search on 'disability rights' and your country name.

Practical tips for study

- Study something you really enjoy!
- Study part time, so the workload is not too much for you.
- Study off campus where possible, use e-lectures, distance education courses, and work from home.
- Register with the student disability support department — their whole reason for being is to help you complete your studies.
- Keep your tutors informed of your progress and your health — they will be glad to help you, and it makes it easier to negotiate extensions or changes to assessments.
- Study in short blocks, when you are well rested, at times that suit you. This is easier to achieve with off campus study.
- Make good use of your campus or local library librarians — they will help you research your assignments and collect information.
- Use technology — iPads, screen readers, dictation software, accessibility settings on your computer and so on — to help you with writing and reading.
- Don't be too hard on yourself if you're not the top of the class — just the fact that you are studying while having this disease is impressive.

Your medical journal

One of the most proactive things you can do is to keep a medical journal. Just get yourself a book with blank lined pages; hardcover is probably best for durability, but a school exercise book will suffice.

Bring it with you to all medical appointments, and take notes either during or immediately after your appointment, while all the details are fresh in your mind.

This notebook is the place to write down your doctors' advice, make notes about medications you're on, record blood and other test results, write down questions to ask as you think of them, track symptoms, write down the details of your next appointment date, and so on. Make sure to date your entries.

You might like to glue the business cards from your specialists and health professionals inside the front cover, so their contact details are always to hand.

These books are a valuable record — your doctors will love that you'll be able to pinpoint the exact date you started on a certain medication or had a certain test done, for example, especially when you have a whole bunch of doctors that you see. They are also a historical document, so you can go back and accurately find out what happened several years before, or when a certain symptom started.

Your medical team

When you have any chronic, complicated, or rare medical condition such as neurosarcoidosis, it's important to gather a supportive medical team. As the patient, you're the head of the team. You're the boss. You're responsible for your own health, with a great team of specialists working for you. Whether it's through your taxes or directly, you are paying them, after all.

On your neurosarcoidosis team you may need some or all of:

- a general practitioner/primary care physician
- an immunologist (immune system specialist)
- a neurologist (nerve specialist)
- a rheumatologist (joint, muscle, ligament specialist)

- an ophthalmologist (eye specialist)
- a dermatologist (skin specialist)
- other specialists if you have sarcoidosis elsewhere
- an occupational therapist or physiotherapist

Never forget that you always have the power to 'hire and fire', even if the pool of options is limited. If, for example, you're really not happy with any particular doctor, try a different one. There are almost always other options, even if it means travelling further, or paying more. It can be a challenge, though, as so few specialists know much about neurosarcoidosis, so your options may be frustratingly limited, depending on where you live.

I know this may not be easy, it may involve more expense, more travel, inconvenience, decision, and delays — but it's *your* health and *your* body after all. It can be very empowering to suddenly realise you *don't* have to keep seeing that dropkick doctor with no people skills who makes you feel two inches tall and tells you your symptoms are all imaginary — you can go elsewhere!

There are wonderful doctors out there who are skilled, knowledgeable, *and* caring human beings to boot. Don't give up.

Getting the most out of medical appointments

You know the experience all too well — you've waited weeks if not months to see your doctor, but after the appointment you feel bewildered, and if anything more confused than before. How can you get the most out of your medical appointments, and find out the information you want to know?

Here are my top 11 tips for how to do this:

1) Make sure any reports from other specialists have been faxed or emailed to your doctor before the appointment; call the office a few days before to check these files have arrived.

2) Make sure that if you need a new referral to your doctor, that you have it ready and with you, or that the referral has been faxed to them before your appointment.

3) If the doctor's office provides a reminder service (phone call, email or text message), sign up for it, so you don't forget appointments. Write them in your diary or calendar. Use reminder alerts on your computer and smart phone. If you need blood tests before your appointment, put in a reminder to have these about a week before your appointment, too, at the same time as you enter the doctor's appointment.

4) Use a medical journal, and write your questions and current or new symptoms in it before you go in to the appointment.

5) Bring a close friend or family member to the appointment if you're having trouble focussing or coping.

6) Have your medical journal open during your appointment, refer to it to jog your memory, and ask your questions one by one. Try to stay on topic.

7) Ask questions of your doctor if anything they say isn't clear to you, ask for more explanation if you need it. It's okay to say 'I don't understand'.

8) Take notes during the appointment of anything your doctor has explained, test results, or anything they're recommending that you do.

9) Ask for copies of blood or other test results, and write the results down, or keep them in a file at home.

10) Ask the following questions when it comes to new treatments:

   • What are my options?

- What are the possible benefits and risks of those options?
- For each option, ask how likely is it that the possible benefits will occur? And how likely are the risks to occur?

11) Remember that you are an important part of your medical team, you're not a passive subject, but an active participant in your own health management.

Personal journals

A private journal is a well-established tool for reducing stress. It allows you to express yourself in a private place, and leave your troubles, fears, and anger on the page rather than racing around and around in your head.

It really does help to write stuff down. Journal-writing has been clinically proven to reduce stress and improve health outcomes[33,34].

You can buy a beautiful blank journal, or use a school exercise book, or a password-protected digital journal program or app such as *Day One* or *Penzu*. If you can, make time to write in your journal for a few minutes every day. Don't worry about your spelling or sentence construction, it's just a safe place where you can get your thoughts down, however that may be. No-one's going to be reading your work!

Some days you might write several pages, others it might just be a couple of words. Sometimes it might be a doodle, a photo, a page full of swear words, or the beginnings of a poem that is forming in your mind ... it's entirely up to you.

Blogs

A blog (short for "we**b log**") is an online diary where you can post photos and diary entries, and other people can leave comments on what you write, if they so desire.

Blogging is generally free; WordPress, Blogger, and Weebly are just a few of the main free blog providers.

When setting up a blog, you can decide on what level of privacy you want — visible to everyone, restricted access to a set of friends who get see it by using a password, or completely private just for yourself. You can also write under a pseudonym, if you wish to maintain your privacy but still have what you write visible to the public.

Running a blog can be a great way to share your experiences with other neurosarcies. You can rant, vent your frustrations, post information you find interesting, whatever you like. It not only helps you, but helps others.

Art therapy

If words are just too hard to put together, it's also very helpful to create drawings and paintings, or even clay sculptures. The goal is to express yourself and your emotions, not to create works of art for display. The act of creation is therapeutic.

What to do:

Gather a few art materials — they can be as simple and inexpensive as a box of coloured pencils, crayons, or some coloured ballpoint pens, or as elaborate as a range of watercolour paints, ink pens, and brushes.

The main thing is to find a medium you like using, and that you won't worry about using up (expensive paints might hamper your style!)

The only other thing you need is something to create your art on — anything with a blank surface will do, from the back of used paper and inexpensive drawing pads, to bound books of watercolour paper and stretched canvas. Art stores sell a wide range of artist's sketchbooks.

To start, find yourself a quiet place and time, when you won't be disturbed, if possible. Take the phone off the hook, turn off your mobile phone. Put on some music that suits your mood.

Think for a few minutes about how you're feeling about your body and neurosarcoidosis. Are you scared? Are you depressed? Angry? Anxious? Feeling isolated?

Choose a colour that represents your mood to you, and start to make marks on the page. You can add words if you like, or even cut pictures out of a magazine and stick them onto your artwork. Cut, draw, glue, scrape, tear. The *activity* of creating is the main focus here, not the end product. You don't need to show it to anyone else. You don't even need to keep it, if you don't want to. You can even burn it.

Music therapy

Another creative therapy is music therapy. Studies have shown that music therapy can help reduce anxiety, pain and depression. It can change physical aspects of your health, like lowering blood pressure, and easing chronic pain[36]. It generally involves working with a professional music therapist, who guides you through such activities as listening to music, guided meditations, singing, whacking a drum, or playing an instrument.

If you search online for 'music therapy' and your region, you will find local resources. And in the mean time, crank up your favourite music, and sing along. Doesn't matter if you can't carry a tune, it's the doing that matters!

Hospitalisation

You may find yourself in hospital now and then with your neurosarc. This section discusses some tips for when you need to go to hospital, and how to manage as well as possible while there.

Ready at a moment's notice

If you're prone to sudden changes in your condition, or recurring serious problems, you may like to have a hospital bag packed in your closet, just in case. Have a change of underwear and some nightwear in it, as well as one or two day's worth of your medication, a notebook and pen, some basic toiletries, ear plugs, and some simple activity you like to do, like a book of puzzles, a favourite magazine or book, or a simple craft project.

Depending on your situation, you may find it useful to write up a summary of your medical history to have in your bag — a basic list of your diagnoses and symptoms, medications, specialists' names and phone numbers, dates of previous admissions, and so on.

Hospital essentials

Hospitals are noisy places that run 24 hours a day. They are not restful. These are some basic things you may like to pack with you, for a hospital stay:

- small notebook and pen
- ear plugs and a sleeping mask
- mobile phone / music player / radio, with earphones and power cords / rechargers
- skin cream and lip balm
- comfortable clothes / nightwear
- a few snacks you enjoy
- enjoyable and easy craft project
- a book or magazine or two

My favourite hospital item is the notebook and pen. With this you can:

- write down what doctors tell you on their rounds
- note down what tests and procedures are done to you, details of any complications or medical advice, and what medication you're on
- make diary entries for each day, and
- vent, rant, and complain in private — whether it's a terse nurse or an impossible room-mate, you can safely get it out of your system in your notebook.

Room–mates

Room-mates can make your stay in hospital more enjoyable (if enjoyable is the right word for being in hospital), or pretty miserable.

The good ...

You can make friends with your room-mates; hospital can be quite lonely (despite being surrounded by people all the time), and having someone in the next bed to chat with makes your stay more pleasant for them and you.

How to be a good room-mate

- The nurse call button makes a noise, so while you should definitely press it when you really need it, continuously pressing it unnecessarily can be annoying.
- Have all your stuff organised and close to hand, keep your area tidy as best you can.
- Wear earphones to listen to music or the TV.
- Ask your visitors to stick to visiting hours, and limit the number who are there at any one time.

- Be conscious of how loud you and your visitors are, try to keep the general noise level down. Stop children from running around too much.

- Treat all hospital staff with courtesy, kindness, and respect, from your surgeon and nurses, to the people who deliver your meals and empty the bins.

- Be patient, sometimes the nurses have more urgent things to do.

- If you are allowed a mobile/cell phone in hospital, keep it on silent or vibration mode, so ringing and alerts don't bother people if you forget to turn it off at night. Talk on the phone quietly.

... and the difficult

There are lots of reasons that people fall into this category — dementia, stroke, fear, non-stop talking, visiting relatives (and whole extended clans), and just plain old difficult personalities. Some are potentially avoidable, others unfortunately not.

If there is a circumstance that can be improved, either ask the patient directly (but politely) or ask the nurses, whichever you feel more comfortable doing — via the nursing staff is likely to be more successful.

Coping with difficult room-mates

- Ear plugs to block out the noise — but do inform the nurses looking after you that you have them in!

- Eye mask to block the light, or to avoid being spoken to.

- Earphones so you can use the radio, music, podcasts, or audiobooks to block out the noise. Listening to music or the TV on earphones can also be relaxing and also means you are not disturbing anyone else. There are some 'sleeping headphone' products available, which are comfortable to sleep in (eg SleepPhones).

- If you aren't in a private room, and want some peace and quiet, pulling the curtains around your bed is a good way of showing that you want some privacy, and one most people understand.

- Keeping a journal. You can complain to your heart's content there! Be careful about people's identities, though, best not to use their actual names.

- Ask the difficult patient's relatives to teach their family member how to use the nurses' call button — it sounds simple and obvious, but is something a surprising number of people struggle to understand.

6

Early symptoms and diagnosis

In this chapter I asked people how long ago they were diagnosed with neurosarcoidosis, and how old they were at the time. What sort of early symptoms did they have, before diagnosis? What led to the diagnosis, and what tests were involved? Who did they see? And what other diagnoses were suggested before neurosarc was decided upon?

I was diagnosed with neurosarcoidosis in March 2012. I was 49 years old. I had never heard of it before my diagnosis.

My early symptoms were fatigue, loss of smell and taste, loss of appetite, weight loss — 30 kg (66 lb) — walking issues (falling over and unsteadiness), eyes closing, double vision, numbness from waist down both legs and feet, numbness of both pinky and ring fingers and half of both hands, and memory loss.

Firstly I went to my GP as I was feeling tired and run down, and at that stage I had lost 10 kg (22 lb). They did blood tests and they came back that I was B12 deficient, so I was given B12 injections for three months as well as daily drops orally. This didn't seem to really help at all. I had other blood tests as I was still feeling run down, and nothing showed up at all.

My regular GP was away, so I went to see another GP as my condition had worsened dramatically — I was starting to fall over without any reason, I was fatigued, had lost over 20 kgs (44 lb), my memory was getting worse, my left eye would close especially when I was tired, and my right eye had double vision. I was struggling to work each day. This GP did some neuro tests on me in the surgery, and suggested I go see a neurologist at our local hospital. I waited for about three months for my appointment, which was in November 2011.

The neurologist did countless examination tests on me during my visit. She had no idea what it could be, but confirmed my symptoms. Multiple sclerosis was mentioned a couple of times. She got the senior neurologist Dr D to come in and confirm her examinations, and asked him what it could be. He thought MS as well. They wanted me to have an MRI, and we booked that in.

Unfortunately the waiting time was quite long and I was too sick to chase it up to get it sooner, so we waited until mid-March 2012 for the MRI. At this stage my condition had really deteriorated. After an episode at work in early March my husband took me to the GP, and suggested that I take some sick leave to get over what I had. The GP gave me till the end of March off on sick leave.

I drove myself to the hospital for the MRI. The MRI took around 50 minutes to do. The nurses told me that I was being taken down to Emergency to be admitted to hospital, and that I would meet my neurologist down there as well.

The neurology registrar was there to meet us. She did numerous prods and pokes on me, went away, then came back with my diagnosis — I was riddled with cancer and had two months to live, if that.

That day I had some fairly horrendous lumbar punctures, and chest x-rays and blood tests. I was admitted to hospital that same day. The next day I had CT scans, some more lumbar punctures and blood tests.

These tests went on for about 10 days, then they decided to do a biopsy through my throat to test a granuloma in my chest to see if it actually tested for cancer or not. A couple of days later my results were in, and no, it was not cancer, but it was neurosarcoidosis.

No one knew much about this condition, but knew that I should get onto steroids straight away. I was on a high dose drip for a full day of steroids then given them orally at 60 mg per day.

I had only seen the neurologist at the stage of diagnosis. A few months later when I went to see my immunologist, he recommended I have a PET scan done so he could get some base markers.

Jill, 51, Australia

I first started to get symptoms of neurosarcoidosis in 1998, when I was 33 years old.

I began having chronic headaches. I was checked for MS, lupus, and migraine and tension headaches. I was sent from one doctor to another, and no one could pinpoint what was going on.

Around 2005 the disease started to progress. I got much more ill, and developed problems with my balance. I walked like a drunken sailor, then I began to pass out, which was extremely worrying. The first time it happened, I was in the car park at my work, about to pick up my son from school. I fell and hit my head — I have no recollection of it happening at all.

As a result of this blackout, I was sent for a CT scan. The doctors discovered some lesions in my brain. But I was still misdiagnosed — including with brain cancer. One doctor even accused me of just wanting pain medications!

In June 2006, I had surgery to put in a shunt near my brain stem. The doctors were sure this would solve all my problems. But my symptoms continued. I was vomiting nearly every day, and staggering when I walked. I started to get vision problems, such as double vision.

After that first blackout, I was given a lot more tests. I was finally referred to Barnes Hospital in St. Louis, where I had 17 days of tests.

In October 2006, the result of a biopsy finally gave me a diagnosis. Neurosarcoidosis.

Kim, 48, USA

I was officially diagnosed with neurosarcoidosis via biopsy on 22 March 2013. I was 42 years old. I believe my symptoms started when I was around my mid-thirties. I developed a lot of burning of my feet at that time during the night that has since then progressed. I also have pulmonary sarcoidosis, and developed **paroxysmal nocturnal dyspnea** around this time.

My symptoms worsened. I developed dizziness shortly after a surgical procedure in 2009. I noticed that the dizziness would get progressively worse. I would get the sensation of being on a roller-coaster or a sinking stomach sensation whenever I was in a car, that I had never experienced before.

I also developed headaches, and a sensation of fogginess in my brain from time to time that would last a couple of hours. It would feel like I was not really present in the moment.

These symptoms progressed in 2011. My headaches were daily, for several months, and located along the frontal area. The dizziness also worsened. I could no longer watch TV as I would get the sensation that I was in an IMAX theater with any sort of movement that I would see on TV. Going to the movie theater would also cause this sensation, that I was moving along with the movie. I noticed it more with any sort of zooming in or out of the camera.

This was followed by getting an MRI of my head, which was negative at that time. I also had a cardiac evaluation done at that time, because I was having twinges of chest pain, but this test was also normal.

Then I developed hearing loss that was bilateral, and tinnitus. I had further development of my neurological symptoms over the following year, with development of a sensation in my left foot of stepping after I had walked a short distance, stopped and was standing. I also developed a warmth and then wet sensation along the outer right lower leg at that time, that was intermittent. This was followed by progressive memory loss, of both new and old memories. I also noticed some difficulty in following and understanding simple commands, and my reading comprehension, and writing skills had also declined since then. I really had to work on processing information that should have been easier to understand.

In January 2013, I developed a ridiculous amount of fatigue, and then fecal incontinence; I went to get this evaluated. The doctor who evaluated me asked if I was having any neurological issues, and then I told him about the symptoms that I had, and he recommended that I see a neurologist. A couple of weeks later, I had a bronchitis-type illness, with severe **arthralgias** and coughing. I went to see a neurologist for my symptoms, and he did an MRI of my brain, neck, and thorax. They noticed four non-specific lesions on my white matter on my brain MRI, and swollen glands in my chest. This was followed up by a CT of my chest, and I was found to have sarcoidosis on my lung lymph biopsy.

I've also had recently a Q-SART test which was positive for small fiber neuropathy.

I have seen my primary care provider, a few neurologists and a few pulmonologists. I also saw a cardio-thoracic surgeon to get the lung biopsy.

I have been diagnosed with migraines as a possibility of the headaches, dizziness, and cognitive fogginess. I was told I was just 'stressed', and was ruled out for multiple sclerosis.

Dr. Farah, 42, USA

I was 35 in 1991 when I first consulted a doctor about neuro symptoms. It was identified as peripheral nerve damage due to sarcoidosis, but it wasn't until 1999 during a flare-up, that the name of neurosarcoidosis was used. I've had sarcoidosis since I was 18, confirmed by eye biopsy.

I think I'd had neurosarc for four years before my diagnosis. I had a baby in 1987 and noticed shooting pains on using hands and flexing feet; when I grasp and turn my hand it's like a shock up my hand and arm. Pins and needles in head, fingers and toes, progressing into face, neck and limbs. Then numbness in my skin and dropping things. I was diagnosed within six months of complaining to my doctor.

So, in summary, I got a positive sarcoidosis diagnosis, by granuloma in eye biopsy in 1986, after 12 years of symptoms. Neuro involvement began and was increasing in 1990. I've not been hospitalised. The tests I had were EMG, X-ray, MRI, lumbar puncture, bloods. My neurologist is my specialist.

I wasn't misdiagnosed with any other diseases. I was told that with neuro problems it is difficult to diagnose until years have gone by, and the symptoms become more obvious. Neuro consultant said that it is possible to have NS and not be able to find granuloma in the brain but that, as I have sarcoidosis, it's probably neurosarc.

Jacqui, 57, Scotland

I was diagnosed with neurosarc in 2002, when I was 53.

I think I had it for three years before getting my diagnosis. In 1999, within a six month period, I had hearing loss with vertigo and tinnitus in my right ear, a left Bell's palsy, then hearing loss in the left ear (no vertigo or ringing).

I had been diagnosed with 'general' sarcoidosis in 1994 after enlarged **hilar nodes** were seen on a chest x-ray (as part of a workup for atrial fibrillation). My lungs were clear and I had no symptoms other than the arrhythmia, which all the doctors said was not sarc-related. So I was not treated and did fine for the next five years, until the hearing loss, etc.

Then in Nov. 2000, a year after the hearing loss and Bell's palsy, I developed sudden severe fatigue and flu-like symptoms, along with severe itching of the eyes (I wanted to scratch my eyelids with a hairbrush). The fever, chills and eye itching improved within a couple of weeks, but the fatigue persisted.

Over the next few months other symptoms appeared, including feeling like I had cobwebs on my face, tremors, balance problems, feet dragging, problems with short-term memory and other cognitive issues.

My PCP tested for mononucleosis (glandular fever), and some other muscle disorders. The tests were all negative, so he concluded that I just needed to spend an hour a day on the treadmill and get more regular sleep! But I was already sleeping in between seeing patients at my prenatal clinic, napping at the nursing station and at the bedside of my laboring moms, as well as napping in my car at the store before driving home, and so on.

Several months later I first saw a neurologist, who immediately suspected neurosarc. I then had a second Bell's palsy, followed by trigeminal neuralgia, both on the left. The neurologist did a bunch more tests, including lumbar puncture, brain MRI, and nerve conduction testing. These were all normal. I had a serum ACE level that was zero, because I'd been on ace-inhibitors for hypertension for years. He really thought it was NS, but was reluctant to treat with the negative test results.

By this time I'd found Dr. S online — he was one of the few NS specialists in the U.S. at that time. There was a midwifery conference coming up in spring of 2002 in the city where he worked, so I got an appointment with Dr S for that week. By the time I saw him, I had developed a severe cough and had my first abnormal chest x-ray, with scattered granulomas and a collapsed right middle lobe. A lung biopsy just before going to see him showed sarc, and the pulmonologist started me on prednisone, 40 mg every other day. After Dr S took a detailed history, did a thorough neuro exam and examined my records, he concluded that there was no doubt I had NS, and recommended prednisone, 40 mg daily. I also started Imuran (azathioprine) a few months later.

In 1994, when I was first diagnosed with sarc, I also had an echocardiogram and pulmonary function tests, which supposedly ruled out sarc involvement in my heart and lungs (other than the nodes). In 1999, when I sustained the hearing loss and Bell's palsy, I saw my PCP, an ENT, and an internist (hallway consultation). None of them picked up on my history of biopsy-proven sarc or connected it to these symptoms.

After the hearing loss in the second ear, I did have an MRI (to rule out MS) and a syphilis test to rule out tertiary syphilis. I also had a test where they put warm and cold water in my ear to see if I puked or got vertigo. Covering the bases there.

In the following years I had tests for mono, rheumatoid arthritis, myasthenia gravis, chronic fatigue (Epstein-Barr), Lyme disease and everything else they could think of. *All* of these test were normal, which is why my PCP told me that I just needed more regular rest/ diet/exercise! But when I started falling out of chairs and having tremors that shook the lunchroom table, I finally requested and got a neuro consult. The neurologist was certain that it was NS, from my medical history and his exam.

But a second MRI was misread as normal here (but abnormal when the films were reviewed by Dr. S a year later). The lumbar puncture he did was also normal (I remember him saying that the protein was slightly elevated, but it was insignificant; years later when I saw another doctor — he looked at my old records and commented that he would have considered it significant.)

This local neuro also did evoked potentials. About that time is when I had a second Bell's palsy, followed by trigeminal neuralgia, both on the left. We discussed treatment with prednisone, either oral or IV pulses, but he wasn't comfortable starting me on the pred train without some positive test results. I was just the second NS patient he'd had (or at least the second one he'd recognized.) I think he was a good doctor and a good neurologist; not perfect, but who is?

So I didn't push for treatment, but did continue research until I found Dr. S, and began an email correspondence that resulted in an appointment with him. It was a 10-hour drive to get to him, so I was able to arrange an appointment with Dr. S for the same week as my midwifery conference (his secretary later told me that he was out of the office that week, but came especially in to see me. There are some dedicated docs out there; it's easy to forget when we run into bozos week in and week out.), so my hotel and airfare were covered by my continuing education money. He spent at least an hour and a half with me, and said the magic words: *'I have no doubt that this is neurosarcoidosis.'*

By the time I went to see Dr S, I'd started respiratory symptoms, seen a lung guy, and had a positive lung biopsy. By the way, the lung doctor told me that I had NS. He said, 'I don't care what the tests say; you have neurosarcoidosis.' *God love him.* The lung guy had started me on 40 mg of pred every other day, but Dr S said neurosarc required daily treatment. He did not do any testing, just reviewed the stack of stuff I took down there.

Other diagnoses I received along the way: poor diet, insufficient exercise, irregular sleep, MS, syphilis, entities unknown.

Rose, 64, USA

I was diagnosed with neurosarcoidosis in September 2011. I was 47 years old. In July 2011, I woke up with some numbness and tingling in my legs. I went to the emergency room and after doing a CT scan, they sent me home with a prescription for prednisone and a referral to an **orthopedic** doctor.

For three weeks I went back and forth, having two MRIs (with and without contrast), and they still did not know what was wrong with me. I also had a CT scan, and a chest x-ray. By this time I needed to use a walker. The orthopedic doctor told me he did not know what was wrong, and that he thought I needed to see a neurologist.

On the first visit, I told the neurologist my symptoms, and he immediately told me that I had **transverse myelitis**, and sent me to the hospital for five days so that I could receive 100 mg of prednisone by IV daily for three days. I got better and returned to work, and was able to walk normal again with physical therapy. I still had some painful muscle spasms, but after three weeks I was finally given the right medicine and dosage and they too went away. I was back to normal by 1 September.

But three weeks later I woke up with the numbness and tingling in my legs, and by night I was totally paralyzed from my waist down, and unable to control my bladder and bowels. I was admitted into the hospital, and spent the next 32 days there before being discharged home, confined to a wheelchair.

A neurologist diagnosed me with neurosarc. I got a second opinion, and he concluded the same diagnosis. Other than transverse myelitis, they thought I had lupus.

Linda, 49, USA

I was diagnosed with neurosarcoidosis in 2009, aged 29.

I think I've had it since I was about 20, when I first started to experience extreme fatigue and then got skin lesions on my legs, so it was nine years before my diagnosis. I had seven years of neurological symptoms (weakness, numbness, tingling, vertigo etc) and five years of uveitis.

In 2009 I had a flare up of symptoms in which I lost my balance and my vision deteriorated, and I was hospitalised to receive IV methylprednisolone. My ophthalmologist suggested to my new neurologist that it may be sarcoidosis (five years after he first said it). (I was previously diagnosed with MS). A new round of tests began.

I had a gallium scan, CT scan (of my chest) and **mediastinoscopy**. My neurologist ordered the first two, and a thoracic surgeon did the biopsy. Prior to that I had numerous MRIs and CTs of the brain. I had also had several lumbar punctures, VERs and EEGs. My ophthalmologist was also involved in the diagnosis.

I saw several neurologists before being diagnosed. Early suggestions of diagnosis included migraine, vasculitis, MELAS (a rare form of dementia) or a psychological cause. I was diagnosed with multiple sclerosis, two years after the neurological symptoms started, even though my ophthalmologist suggested sarcoidosis at this time. I was treated for MS for five years, before being officially diagnosed with sarcoidosis/neurosarcoidosis.

Leah, 34, Australia

I was diagnosed with sarcoidosis in 2005 at the age of 25, and neurosarcoidosis in 2007 at the age of 27. I suspected that something was bad wrong since I was 16, but no one really wanted to listen to me. My first really strange symptom was at 18 after I was newly married. I woke up one morning and went to the bathroom like I did every morning. I tried to urinate and was not able to. I had lost the ability to do so for no reason.

My husband took me to the ER and they thought that I had a urinary tract infection. They gave me some antibiotics, inserted a catheter and sent me home for a couple days. I returned a few days later, had the catheter removed, and expected to be able to urinate. A few hours later I returned to the ER, and had to have the catheter put back in place because I could not urinate. After weeks of doing this and seeing a urologist, no reason was determined and no infection was ever found. But after about two months, as quickly as I has stopped urinating, the urge came back. I later would learn it was one of the first signs of my autonomic system being attacked by the neurosarcoidosis.

My neurosarcoidois diagnosis came after my sarcoid continued to progress, and I kept having strange symptoms that made no sense. Along with the dizziness, heart palpitations, strange pupil changes, electric shock feelings, tingling and numbness, I also was having very low blood pressure readings — 80/40 was a normal reading for me, and I had begun to faint frequently. I had also lost the ability to feel hot things especially, and had burnt myself on many occasions with the stove and bath water, so my husband knew something was wrong. We mentioned it to Dr. P at the Cleveland Clinic when I went for my usual sarc apt. He then sent me to a neurologist, who set me up for neurological testing. I went for autonomic nerve testing, and I also had nerve biopsy testing along with a spinal tap, EMG, CT and MRI of my brain and spine.

Other diagnoses that were considered were multiple sclerosis and stage 4 lymphoma.

Andrea, 34, USA

I was given a 'possibly neurosarcoidosis' diagnosis in September 2010, when I was 46. Over the months it became clearer that neurosarc was the best diagnosis, so now it's a '99% definitely NS' diagnosis (just missing a tissue biopsy for 100% confirmation). I appear to have the relapsing-remitting type of neurosarc, so I have long times when the disease is well-controlled, with occasional severe flares.

I've had weird but minor neurological and autoimmune symptoms on and off since 2003, but no-one really took any notice, as everything was mild and nonspecific. I had phantom sensations on my feet, like a piece of sticky tape was on my toes, and my senses of smell and taste 'faded out' once or twice a year (and thankfully faded back in). I also had tender areas, crippling fatigue, foot pain, brain fog, and insomnia. I was diagnosed with fibromyalgia / chronic fatigue.

In 2005 I had a sixth nerve palsy (causing severe double vision), which put me in hospital, but they couldn't figure out what caused it. My lumbar puncture at the time was normal, and the palsy slowly got better by itself. My vision hasn't been that great since then, my eyes are prone to going blurry from fatigue very quickly, and they get very dry.

In September 2010 I lost about a third of my vision in both eyes overnight, and developed numbness around my mouth, and down my right arm. This put me in hospital for three weeks in all, and got me the diagnosis of 'possibly NS'. On the day I left hospital they finally started me on prednisolone. Frustratingly, I didn't receive any other treatment while I was in hospital, although the blindness was progressing over that time.

I had a lumbar puncture, which was initialy misread as normal, but was actually abnormal (oligoclonal bands and increased white blood cells). I've also had CT scans, MRIs with and without contrast (the MRI with contrast showed up the lesions around the optic chiasm), and tons of neurological and blood tests.

They didn't do any of the more invasive tests like a cerebral angiogram as I've had a **pulmonary embolism** before (after hip surgery), and I have a high risk of developing blood clots.

Other diagnoses I've had along the way have been fibromyalgia and/or chronic fatigue. After my vision loss, MS and vasculitis were also considered.

Denise, 50, Australia

I was diagnosed in 1997, 16 years ago. I was 44 years of age. I had first symptoms in my eyes in 1993.

They thought it was **Ménière's disease**. I was scheduled for surgery for my ears when I really got bad and couldn't function at all. I couldn't understand how to put my pants on, because the pants had one hole and I had two legs. I was rushed to hospital.

The **ventricle** in my brain swelled shut, which caused the brain to swell with fluids. They were trying to find out what was causing everything, and they admitted me into the hospital for exploratory surgery, but then the ventricle exploded in the front part of my head, before I even got to the surgery room. I was shaking all over, couldn't remember anything for even five minutes and had terrible vertigo. They inserted a temporary shunt into the ventricle in the brain, right there in the prep room, and drained it into a bag until they could figure out what was wrong.

I spent hours in CT scans. They sent my brain fluid to Mayo Clinic. Neurosarcoidosis was suspected, and they took a lung biopsy to get the diagnosis.

Ménière's disease, lupus, MS, and brain tumors were also considered before I got the diagnosis of neurosarc.

Kathleen, 60, USA

I was diagnosed with neurosarcoidosis in June 2012. I was 26 years old. The more I think about it, I think I may have had it since my early 20s. But it was around January 2012 right up until May where a multitude of issues started to come to the surface. These included chronic headaches, night sweats, dizziness, vomiting, toilet and bladder issues, erectile dysfunction due to deteriorated testosterone levels, sudden weight loss, occasional speech impediment, and strange sharp pains in my head. I knew there was something wrong but never thought all the symptoms were linked as they were so varied.

In early May 2012, I had a particularly bad episode where I got a really severe headache and felt dizzy, so I sat down and waited for my girlfriend. When she arrived I tried to speak but the words came out really jumbled and she could not understand me. My mouth was also drooping to one side — she thought I was having a stroke.

She made me go to the doctor who was shocked by my condition and sent me to the A+E department in the hospital. After waiting for many hours I was eventually seen and they did a multitude of tests including CT scans and blood tests. They came to the conclusion that I suffered from migraines, gave me sufficient medication to treat it for three days and sent me home.

Needless to say, my issues did not go away, in fact they got worse. Over the next few weeks my issues worsened and in particular my walking. I seemed to walk as if I was drunk staggering from side to side, and there was nothing I could do about it.

On 22 May I went for a walk into town — halfway there I didn't feel right, so I sat down on a nearby wall. After a few minutes I tried to stand back up but I wasn't able to. I thought about ringing someone, but the battery in my phone had died. Eventually I managed to struggle back to my girlfriend's house, holding onto walls along the way. I made it, and a hour later we were back at the doctor. He was angry that I had been sent home from the hospital weeks earlier, as he knew it was more complex than just migraines, and wrote a letter to ensure that I was kept in overnight for tests. That was the beginning of a 29 day stay in hospital.

I underwent many tests over the weeks that followed including two lumbar punctures, two bronchoscopies, MRIs, CT scans and had physiotherapy daily; I walked with a crutch for the next three months. The doctors I saw were from the neurology and endocrinology departments, including a lung doctor who was a sarcoidosis specialist.

Other diseases that were suggested as possibilities for me were tuberculosis and lymphoma. In fact I was put on TB medication for many months as a precaution.

Percy, 27, Ireland

7
Symptoms

In this chapter I asked people what their current symptoms of neurosarcoidosis are.

I have numbness, stiffness and weakness in my legs. Soreness, tightness, and burning in my back that wraps around to my chest.

I have trouble sleeping. I wake up every two to three hours. I'm unable to sleep on my side because of the paralysis, I can't turn from side to side.

My legs seem really heavy after sitting for more than an hour. I have numbness from my waist down. I have some feeling but not all. I can't determine if something is cold or hot from my waist down. I'm incontinent, too.

Linda, 49, USA

Early on my symptoms included chronic headaches, night sweats, difficulty walking, dizziness, vomiting, toilet and bladder problems, erectile dysfunction, sudden weight loss, and occasional speech impediments. Thankfully some of those issues have been resolved — I don't suffer from the headaches any more, and my testosterone levels are back to normal thanks to applying Testogel daily for four months following my hospitalization.

The main unresolved issues are permanent damage to my right leg due to the scarring on my brain, this affects my walking, and limits my ability to do certain exercises and movements, and I can't play sports.

The toileting issues also have not been resolved; about a month ago I spent the night in hospital to under go a deprivation test but even that could not determine what the problem was.

Percy, 27, Ireland

My current NS symptoms ("residuals" since the NS is presumably in remission) are:
Bilateral hearing loss
Problems with balance
Vertigo when looking up or lying flat
Disorientation as to where I am
Problems with short term memory, focus and concentration
Poor word recall (has worsened in recent years)
Peripheral neuropathy, especially in feet (has worsened over the years)
Residual pain left side of face and eye from trigeminal neuralgia
Secondary **Sjögren's syndrome**
Fatigue
Muscle weakness and cramps
Tremors
Choking on liquids

Other weird symptoms:
Sudden jerks of a leg or foot
Shivers in odd places on the body
Feeling of vibration, like a pager, on the back and legs
Feeling like my whole body was shaking, but wide awake and able to move —nothing like a seizure (the first time I thought it was an earthquake when I woke up — we do have them in Indiana occasionally.)

Major problems:

Feet. Numbness — sometimes can't feel pedals when driving. But, it hurts to press on pedals with balls of feet. Hurts to wear shoes, sandals. But, it hurts to walk on carpet without shoes or slippers. Hurts to have feet even slightly cool. Carry blankets everywhere to wrap up feet.

Plus frequent squeezing pain. Toes pull up way far; can't move toes. Can't stand to touch them when this happens. Warm water helps slightly. Mostly just have to wait it out; sometimes a couple of hours or more. Often can't bend feet at toes; hard to get up from floor. Can only stand for a few minutes.

Muscle weakness. Right arm gets tired just cutting up a fried egg. Carrying wallet in either hand makes hands and arms very tired.

Painful hands. Wake up feeling like tight clenched fists all night. They ache all day, worse if I close my fingers; have to hold steering wheel loosely, even with padded steering wheel. Use foam on pen.

Focus and memory. I cannot focus on any activity needing a brain for more than a few minutes. It takes me a day or two to read the Sunday paper. I can't read books because I have to keep starting over or take notes, which I can't figure out. When I try to pay bills or do a budget, after a few minutes I can't remember what the checkmarks or stars mean, why I highlighted something. I just sit, paralyzed, trying to figure out what I was doing. I really need someone to take over my financial affairs, but there isn't anybody.

It takes me hours to do what I used to do in a few minutes. I'm still writing notes to myself like 'Cut nails' on Post-it notes, TV guides, church bulletin, but the notes just crawl under papers and other stuff. I don't even remember writing them, even when it's something very important. Like paying my neurologist.

Rose, 64, USA

Memory loss

Mobility issues — cannot drive any more. Need a walker to walk around house, use a wheelchair or scooter for outside of house.

Balance issues, cannot stand for very long

Bladder issues (self catheterising 3 x daily)

Numbness of legs and feet and severe pain in feet

Numbness of pinky and ring fingers on both hands and also half of hands as well

Loss of taste and smell

At times smelling things that aren't there — like smoke or faeces

Severe weight gain from steroids + 40 kg (88 lb)

Oesteoarthritis, from steroids. Have fractured L1 in back.

Lack of interest in anything

No concept of time

Pains in joints and back pain

Lots of other aches and pains in different areas

Noticeable lesions in arms, legs, neck, and shoulder areas

Got blood clot in August 2012 in my leg

Jill, 51, Australia

Skin lesions, starting at ankles and spreading up to waist and arms

Neurological symptoms — vertigo, numbness and tingling (pretty much everywhere at some point), facial numbness, blurred vision, double vision

Difficulty speaking

Mood fluctuations

Loss of strength and balance

Bladder dysfunction

Cognitive processing problems and short term memory loss

Severe fatigue

Chest pain

Severe uveitis

Nausea

Leah, 34, Australia

I currently have profound fatigue, headaches, dizziness, loss of hearing, tinnitus, decreased taste, bright flashes in my left eye, with an occasional black central spot, bloody nostril on the left (learned this may be due to the small fiber neuropathy causing excessive dryness of the nasal mucosa). I also have cognitive decline, where my IQ has declined 36 points; memory loss, and inability to multi-task or to do basic arithmetic. I have left side numbness of my face and lips, dry mouth, loss of taste, stuttering, numbness of my hands and fingers, decreased grip strength of my right hand, warm/wet sensation in my lower legs, loss of stool intermittently, and burning of my feet.

I have severe shortness of breath, palpitations, chest pain, cold intolerance, jitteriness, and frequent episodes of feeling faint which is all due to autonomic dysfunction from the sarcoidosis. My cardiologist told me that I am at very high risk for sudden death due to my recurrent episodes of passing out, and the severity of my shortness of breath.

Dr Farah, 43, USA

Small patch of blindness in one eye, central. It still annoys me, after years. Occasional numbness in my face, or phantom sensations like there's a piece of hair caught on my eyelid. Some peripheral neuropathy in my hands and feet. **Paraesthesia** (pins and needles, numbness) in my right arm at times. Occasional **dysesthesia** on my limbs. I usually feel cold, even on a hot summer's day, and don't seem to sweat much. Food intolerances, which are a new thing for me — salicylates and amines in particular.

I periodically lose my sense of smell and taste; they usually 'fade' back in after a month or so, but they have been worse in recent times, and not recovering as well. Sometimes I can only taste sweet and salty things on one side of my tongue. Occasional phantom smells. Onycholysis.

Melkersson-Rosenthal syndrome (granulomas in the lips causing them to swell, temporarily, and facial numbness). Mildly abnormal liver blood tests and possible liver involvement. Used to get horrible raised red itchy lesions on my lower legs, but they haven't come back since I've been on immune suppressants. Foot pain. Headaches.

Denise, 50, Australia

Short term memory loss, some small tremors. Balance issues. Headaches, loss of hearing. The headaches are so bad that I can't even sit up in bed. Vertigo, eyes bleeding in the back of the eye. Fatigue, ringing of the ears, chest pains, wheezing, dry cough.

Kathleen, 60, USA

My symptoms include dizziness, blackouts, slurred speech, vision problems, headaches, vomiting, and loss of balance — I have to use a walker to get around, cannot balance without it.

Kim, 48, USA

Severe headache at back of head and down spine to lumbar area. Exhaustion, sleepiness, dizziness, walking to one side, can't do two things at once — i.e. walking at the same time as talking. Nausea on exertion, stinging eyes, sore throat, blurred vision, light and noise sensitivity; tingling and numbness in limbs, face head and neck; memory loss, confusion, concentration problems, tinnitus; swollen face, breasts and glands; twitching muscles, cramps in legs and feet, parasomnia, dyscalculia, aphasia, lucid dreams, insomnia, temperature control problems — freezing and unable to warm up one minute, then roasting the next.

Jacqui, 57, Scotland

I have numbness and tingling in my legs, feet, arms, hands, torso, and face like a mask. I have a burning sensation that is constant in the back of my head and I have twitching in both of my lower eyelids that is not simultaneous, but is constant even at rest.

My right eye has much worse vision loss than the left eye, and I have a constant ringing in my ears that gets worse the sicker I am. I also get electric shocks, especially in my left arm and down my right leg. I have a burning pain like a hot poker that radiates up my right foot like someone is sticking a hot poker to the bottom of my foot. I have severe pain reduction from the knees down and elbows down when it comes to sharp objects and heat, and have hurt myself unknowingly many times.

I still have problems with my bladder and bowels. I urinate constantly, like 20 times some days, and barely urinate other days. I have diarrhea some days and can have constipation the next — this is caused by the sarcoidosis attacking the autonomic system.

My body also does not have the ability to regulate temperature anymore so I can be literally freezing cold on a 90°F (32°C) day, and burning up when it is cold. I really have to try to pay attention to what my body is telling me, because I usually don't sweat so I can overheat very easy on a hot day.

I now have a defibrillator/pacemaker to help protect me from sudden cardiac death for two reasons. I have cardiac sarcoidosis which can cause heart related problems, but I also have autonomic dysfunction and that causes low blood pressures, shortness of breath. Because I have poor circulation, this causes a greater risk of heart related problems and sudden cardiac death as well.

So far my sarcoidosis has been found in my eyes, skin, saliva glands, heart, lungs, lymph nodes, liver, spleen, pancreas, kidneys, bone marrow, terminal ileum, spine, and nervous system including small fiber and autonomic.

Andrea, 34, USA

8
Management and treatment

In this chapter, I asked how people's neurosarcoidosis is managed, and what treatments they're on. What sort of doctors do they see? What sorts of regular tests for monitoring disease activity do they have? How does the medication affect them?

I have unsuccessfully been on prolonged, high dose prednisone, methotrexate, Neurontin and plaquenil. The long term steroids caused me to develop the inevitable, Cushingoid syndrome, with a 40 lb (18 kg) weight gain. Methotrexate caused severe nausea, and vomiting. The Neurontin gave me suicidal thoughts, and I developed **methemoglobinemia** [a blood disorder that leads to less oxygen in the body] from the Plaquenil, so they had to be stopped.

Currently, I am on Remicade (infliximab), CellCept (mycophenolate mofetil), Imuran (azathioprine), atenolol, and a topical compound for my neuropathy. We are trying to start **IVIG** for my **dysautonomia** [malfunctioning of the autonomic nervous system] however, it is extremely difficult to get insurance approval for this medicine as it is an off label use for the drug.

Of the medication that I am on currently, I have only noticed some relief of my joint pains with the Remicade, and the atenolol has controlled my heart rate. With these medicines, I still feel like I am only 20% of the person that I was before getting ill.

I have seen my primary care physician, pulmonologists, neurologists, and a rheumatologist, ophthalmologist and cardiologist. I have also had to work with speech, physical and occupational therapists. It took me a very long time to find a healthcare team that I was comfortable with. I sought out "specialists" in sarcoid by looking up who published recent medical articles of neurosarcoidosis. However, my physicians helped me find other specialists that completed my healthcare team successfully.

The most difficult physicians I found were neurologists. I had to go through several of them. My experiences with them were that they were dismissive, and failed to do the necessary tests. I think several of the physicians that I encountered were overwhelmed by the multiple symptoms that I was presenting with.

Dr Farah, 43, USA

I currently have an injection of methotrexate (25 mg) once a week. I also use Prednefrin Forte and Combigan eye drops for uveitis. I take other medications for symptoms as necessary such as Ditropan for bladder dysfunction, ondansetron for nausea, and Panadeine Forte for pain.

Major flare ups of symptoms are usually treated with doses of IV methylprednisolone or injections of steroids under the eye.

After a significant flare up last year I required several weeks in a rehabilitation hospital.

In the past I have tried Imuran (azathioprine), methotrexate (orally), and CellCept (mycophenolate mofetil). I also tried cyclophosphamide (chemotherapy).

I also manage my sarc by trying to eat well and get exercise, I go to the gym and work with a personal trainer. This exercise program has greatly improved my ability to walk. I try and get plenty of rest and find ways to minimize stress, as that can have a big impact on my symptoms. I also see a psychologist when the disease overwhelms me.

My medical team is my neurologist, ophthalmologist, rheumatologist and my GP.

I think they do the best they can with a complicated and misunderstood disease. My GP provides me more with support than treatment, and got me through the very rough year in which I was re-diagnosed (from MS to neurosarc).

My ophthalmologist is fantastic but his focus is on the uveitis, and subsequent increased pressure and cataracts (which have now been removed, and intraocular lenses have been inserted).

My neurologist probably has the most difficult task. He did re-diagnose me and for that I am grateful, but we go around in circles a lot because to date none of the immunosuppressant drugs have been effective; however the methotrexate injections have been promising.

I see a rheumatologist to manage the use of the methotrexate as it needs to be monitored due to side effects. I also have an injection nurse at my GP's clinic to give me the injection.

I have been fortunate that the methotrexate injection has not given me any problems as far as side effects go, because many of the other options had. I have had significant weight gain from years of methylprednisolone.

Leah, 34, Australia

At the moment my sarcoidosis is managed by a Remicade infusion every eight weeks, and 750 mg CellCept twice daily. I have reacted well to both medications, and I am very happy with how my recuperation has gone.

Initially I was put on a cycle of steroids to reduce the inflammation on my brain. I was innocent and clueless about what effects this medication would have on me. The effects soon became clear: weight gain, increased appetite, sleeplessness, and it made my facial features puffy. This was quite hard for me as a young, relatively vain male. I gained 19.5 kilos (43 lb) in the three months that followed, I went from 75 (165 lb) to 94.5 kilos (208 lb) at my heaviest. I went from being too thin to fat in a very short time.

Percy, 27, Ireland

I am currently being managed with intravenous immunoglobulin (IVIG) treatments, and narcotics for the pain. I have failed treatment with prednisone, leflunomide, Plaquenil, Imuran, Remicade, CellCept, and methotrexate. I am waiting to see if I am a candidate for **allogenic** stem cell transplant at Northwestern University Chicago. My doctors at Cleveland say I only have Rituxan and **plasmapheresis** left to try. The Rituxan would help my overall sarcoidosis if it works, and the plasmapheresis would help my failing autonomic system that, if left untreated, eventually will cause me to lose limbs, due to no circulation — or my life. Both treatments have great risk involved.

My medical team consists of: neurologist, pulmonologist, sarcoidosis specialist, endocrinologist, pain management specialist, ophthalmologist, gastroenterologist, headache specialist, **electrophysiologist**, cardiologist, oncologist, and urologist.

Andrea, 34, USA

I've lost count of the number of MRIs and spinal taps I've had. I am undergoing chemotherapy (Cytoxan (cyclophosphamide) every 90 days), which I have in the hospital. I take prednisone every day (I'm down to 10 mg/day, after starting on 60 mg). I take pain meds as needed, and Ativan for nervous times. I take spirolactone to control swelling.

My face is puffy and swollen from the steroids. My eyes water all the time. My speech is sometimes slurred because of occasional paralysis on one side of my mouth. I have lost my hair from the chemo treatment.

Kim, 48, USA

In 2006, after almost four years of immune suppressants, I was considered in remission of both my neuro and pulmonary sarc.

Then in 2011 I was diagnosed with cardiac sarc, but we could find no indication of active sarc anywhere else in my body, either by testing or by symptoms. I talked it over with my heart and lung guys, and decided to get an implanted pacemaker/defibrillator, but hold off on the very high-dose prednisone recommended for cardiac sarc. I was remembering the 90 lb (40 kg) weight gain from my first go round with pred.

Things were fine for another year, until I had a lung flare, with some new granulomas popping up in my lungs. So last year I restarted the pred at 40 mg/day and Imuran 50 mg 3x/day.

I've actually lost weight this time, I imagine because this time I developed insulin-dependent diabetes! I've done well with the diabetes, most of the time.

But my blood pressure's got all out of whack this year, requiring at one time four anti-hypertensives to keep it under control. Then I got septic from a UTI, which triggered **atrial fibrillation**. All that actually lowered my blood pressure, and now I'm on three meds for blood pressure, but one of those is also for the **arrhythmia**.

Through all this heart and lung mess, my neuro status has remained stable. The fatigue is much worse these past few months, but I'm sure that's related to the heart/lung stuff. My hearing in my right ear has deteriorated a bit this last year, but I saw my ENT, and he could find no evidence that sarcoidosis was involved; he thinks it is age-related.

The meds I'm on right now for neurosarc stuff: prednisone and Imuran for lung sarc, but might scare the neuro nasties away too; Lyrica, nortripyline (for peripheral neuropathy, and an anti-depressant); Restasis eye drops, Klonopin, and insulin and extra blood pressure meds thanks to pred.

To help me cope, I have comfort measures for neuropathic pain, hearing aids, and am learning speech reading. I get other people to change light bulbs, and watch my surroundings — terrain, walls or rails. I use a walker and scooter as needed, and follow up with my health care team as needed.

My specialists:

Internal medicine specialist or his nurse practitioner (NP) for primary care

Pulmonologist/sarc specialist for lungs and general sarc management Local neurologist for routine follow-up, and if I have any new or troubling symptoms

Cardiologist/electrophysiologist and his NP for the cardiac sarc

Psychiatrist for the depression and to manage the Ritalin (for ADHD).

I have no problems working with any of them; they or a staff member have always been available when I needed them. When my neuro first saw me and told me he believed that I had NS (only his second case), he knew a little more than I did about it. But within a few months, I had learned so much, and he has always been open and receptive to what I've wanted to share with him. He encourages me to have an endpoint goal, and looks at pluses and minuses to get there.

My other docs have similar philosophies, although the cardiologist is a bit more withdrawn, and I won't pretend to know more than he does about cardiac sarc! But even with him, when he recommended the implantable cardioverter-defibrillator (AICD), he explained his rationale, but didn't give me any grief when I decided to think about it for a few months.

Rose, 64, USA

I currently use azathioprine (Imuran), acupuncture, Beconase, tramadol, capsaicin, and diclofanac sodium gel. I have monthly blood tests for being on azathioprine. Bone density scans.

My neurologist is an inflammatory specialist and good at supporting me, but I don't know if he really understands neurosarc. He's now off long-term sick himself, and there's no actual sarcoid specialist in our area. So, as I'm having new problems, my GP is sending me to the nearest neurologist. I'm concerned that this doctor has no mention of NS or sarcoidosis on his CV. My GP is reluctant to send me to the sarcoid clinic in England, as we live in Scotland, but as far as I know there's no clinic specialising in NS here.

I don't feel my GP listens to me, as I've often asked if new symptoms are sarcoid related, and he said that it wouldn't matter as I'm already being treated for sarcoid, and any new symptoms will pass!

Prednisolone had many side effects including hair loss, weight gain and brain symptoms, but it's hard to separate them from the sarcoid symptoms — reducing steroids means I get fewer side effects, but the steroids also help reduce my sarc symptoms. No obvious side effects from azathioprine. Though it does modify the disease, the nerves haven't completely healed and I still get flare-ups.

Jacqui, 57, Scotland

I can no longer work, so am at home now. I try to do some physio exercises at home when I am well enough, as there are still days where I just cannot get out of bed.

I am still having bladder issues. Just had a urinary tract infection which made me incontinent.

I get regular INR (international normalised ratio) blood tests from the nurses at my GP, to check how I'm going on the warfarin.

I am getting infusion of infliximab (Remicade) every eight weeks, which I find helps me with my balance and feeling better. Helps with sore joint pain as well. I have one infusion left, and we have to apply to the Medical Board to see if I can get some more.

I am on CellCept (mycophenolate mofetil), prednislone, Bactrim, OxyContin, Lyrica, a vitamin D tablet and warfarin.

I see a rheumatologist and she is wonderful and mainly prescribes my drugs. She is the one who pushed for me to be on CellCept and get the infusions with the Medical Board.

I see an immunologist, and he has studied sarcoidosis so it's good, and I have found that he is very good with reviewing my treatment. I also see a neurologist. He just does a check up with me now and then for review.

I was seeing an ophthalmologist as I was going blind in the left eye, which is all good now. I see a haematologist for the blood clot, and an endocronologist as because of the steroids I am on the brink of getting diabetes, so he is monitoring this.

I find that the rheumatologist, immunologist, and neurologist have discussions about my condition in a patient type of meetings. I always make sure that each of the three specialists above are all advised of any tests that I get done, or if I am in hospital again.

I have monthly blood tests, and a regular MRI — around every six months now.

Steroids: Positives; it suppresses symptoms to help with every day life Negatives; weight gain, getting osteoarthritis, and borderline diabetes.

Methotrextrate: Didn't do anything. Negatives; loss of hair, lesions doubled in size when I was on this and cyclophosphamide.

Most effective for me was the CellCept. It has helped clear my mind and help me think again. I can now string a sentence now, whereas before I could not do this. This drug has bought me back into the land of the living — prior to this I cannot remember anything much at all.

When I was on Endone it was good for pain relief, but I think I was a bit of a nutter on it too!

Jill, 51, Australia

I'm on Imuran (azathioprine) once a day, and Baclofen, OxyContin, and gabapentin each three times a day.

I started seeing a new neurologist recently. The one I was seeing prior to him was not friendly or personable. He made me feel that he was too busy for my questions.

I have regular complete blood count blood tests. My results are lower than what my doctor wants, which is why I only take one dose of Imuran daily. My normal dose is three times a day.

How does the medication affect me? I'm just so tired. I want to sleep more. I guess the Imuran works because the inflammation has not come back. The gabapentin I take for the soreness is not working. Prior to the gabapentin, I tried Lyrica and that did not work either.

Linda, 49, USA

I have the remitting form of neurosarc, with flares and periods of disease remission. So when I'm in remission I don't require such aggressive medical treatment for the sarc.

When I was first diagnosed, I was put on prednisolone at 60 mg/day. Tapered down gradually over 11 months. Then I was on methotrexate and azathioprine (Imuran), but my liver reacted badly to them, so

I had to move on to mycophenolate mofetil (CellCept). I still take CellCept every day (currently tapering down), and a vitamin D supplement, as I'm deficient.

I see my GP, immunologist, and ophthalmologist regularly, every three to nine months. I see a liver specialist once a year, and my neurologist and dermatologist when I need to. My latest addition to the gang is a dietician.

I have a brain MRI with contrast once a year or so, to see how things are going. I have blood tests before every immunology appointment, and do visual field tests every time I see my ophthalmologist too. I've had a few nerve conduction studies, various other scans, and several lumbar punctures.

When I was on prednisolone, I gained 19 kg (42 lb), had steroid-induced diabetes, manic behaviour (when taking high doses), insomnia, heartburn, easy bruising and so on. Highly unpleasant — but it *did* work, took me from ~40% vision loss in both eyes to 13% loss in only one eye, which is now only 8% loss (it's been improving slowly, even since I've been off the pred).

I seem to tolerate the CellCept pretty well. It does give me intermittent nausea and diarrhoea. Still, much better than the pred!

In recent times I have developed a lot of food intolerances (which my dietician says can develop in autoimmune disease like sarcoidosis and if you're on immune suppressants). I'm on a very strict and restrictive diet now — the Royal Prince Alfred Hospital food intolerance diet. It avoids salicylates, amines and glutamates: **www.sswahs.nsw.gov. au/rpa/allergy/resources/foodintol/**. It's also known as the Failsafe diet. This has helped to reduce many of my 'chronic fatiguey' sorts of symptoms. My brain fog, mood, sleep and fatigue are vastly improved, so it's proving to be worth the considerable pain of the diet! Frankly, this book wouldn't have been finished without it.

Denise, 50, Australia

Currently I take 10 mg of prednisone every day. Was up to 120 mg of steroids at one time. Tried three times to lower from 10 mg, and always end up having my brain swell and needing more surgery. The doctors I see are GP, rheumatologist, neurosurgeon, and an eye specialist.

I have regular tests. I've been having brain scans every six months because the right side of my brain is swollen again. I see my rheumatologist every three to six months.

Kathleen, 60, USA

9
Life impact

In this chapter I asked people how neurosarcoidosis has affected their family and social life. What about work and studies? And have they been able to access any sort of government support?

This disease can take a very heavy toll on our lives. My informal, unscientific and very small survey showed that roughly half of people with neurosarc are so affected by the disease they're unable to work or study. In round figures:

> 20% are able to work or study full time

> 30% are able to work or study from home

> 50% unable to work or study*

* Poll run on the neurosarcoidosis group on Facebook in June 2013, 28 respondents. 6 working or studying full time; 5 studying from home; 3 working from home; 14 unable to work or study.

I had to move home when I got sick, and I rely on my immediate family for a lot of support. It's tough being a young person who has to move home and become dependent on parents again, but I'm grateful that they help me.

Fatigue plays a big part of how much I can do. Not being able to drive anymore is very frustrating. I think my friends understand, but I also think they get frustrated and/or bored with me being sick. Sometimes it can be very hard to say no and when you do you feel guilty, but I can't always keep up. I lost a lot of friends when I got sick, and some of my extended family tends to stay away.

The mood fluctuations caused by the neurosarc also have an impact on my relationships with friends, family and even colleagues. I have no control over them and this can be one of the most upsetting symptoms.

I have not been in paid employment since the neurological symptoms started, despite several efforts to return. I do volunteer work, but find this exhausting some times. I also study part time. With both volunteering and study I require frequent rest breaks and adaptive technology for my low vision.

I am grateful to be on the Australian Disability Support Pension.

Leah, 34, Australia

I've a very supportive and understanding close family. I exist by pacing and resting, depending on how ill I am. I can achieve many things when given no time limit, and can look quite well at times, but my family is always concerned and warn me when I begin to look tired. When I'm having a really bad spell, I'm unable to get up and about, so I am literally hibernating until I begin to feel better. That stage can go on for months and years.

At my best, I can attend a social event, if I rest all day before going out. I have been able to attend a whole wedding by booking a room at the hotel, and excusing myself for a few hours during the day to go and rest. I've had sarcoid most of my life (since I was 18), so friends and family are aware of my instability and possible restrictions I have to make. At first I couldn't explain why I was so ill, and some relatives didn't give me the credibility I should have had. Once I was diagnosed, it was better, but then I didn't want to say how ill I really was.

I was able to work until my sarcoid became neurosarc. Then my employers did everything they could to keep my job open for two years, but I couldn't get well enough to go back. My good days are so limited and I can't predict how long a good spell will last, that I can't realistically take on work.

I did think that if I was my own boss, I could choose when to work, but my business idea fell through due to me being too ill.

I went to tribunal and was awarded Employment and Support Allowance. I am in the support group so I don't have to attend work related interviews. I've had DLA (Disability Living Allowance) in the past when appropriate, after winning tribunals, which I relinquished on improving.

Jacqui, 57, Scotland

I don't have the energy to take care of my house and yard like I used to. My family helps, but they all work and have family themselves. I used to play guitar and do crafts like cross stitch, but I've had to give that up. I can still crochet and macramé, and I help my grandkids do simple crafts. I watch more TV than I should. It's just such a production to get settled in my chair with my feet up and cozy, that I wait as long as possible to leave my little nest!

I don't have much social life outside my family and online buddies. Most of my friends were work friends, and I when I had to quit work it became difficult to get together with them. We still talk occasionally, but I miss our girls' nights out. I have some church friends, but I don't go to church as much as I used to because it's such a hassle to get my walker out and find a place to sit where I can read the pastor's lips. They have a pretty good sound system, but I still miss a lot of what's said.

I miss my old friends; we say that we need to get together, but it just doesn't happen. There is a group of retired nurses that meets for breakfast once a month. I've gone a couple of times, but there are usually at least eight or nine of them, and I just can't understand what they are saying most of the time, so it makes me feel more isolated to sit in a group of people, laughing away, and I have no idea what they are saying. I'd rather have my pity parties at home, with my dogs, cats, and Judge Judy!

When I first lost my hearing, I got hearing aids and went on working, but I had difficulty hearing, especially on the phone or with a lot of background noise. Hospitals, especially nursing stations, are just noisy, but it drove me nuts, worrying about what important info I might miss. I did buy some portable phone amplifiers that you strap on to the phone. Those helped a lot. The hospital bought a special stethoscope that enabled me to hear heart and lung sounds. Those things got me through a couple of years, until the fatigue and neuropathy began to get bad.

I made it through another year, until the cognitive and respiratory issues, along with the muscle weakness, brought it to an end. My feet hurt so bad by the end of the day that I wanted to cry. I was stressed out from the strain of trying to hear all day. I was at the hospital late every night finishing my charting because I had so much trouble remembering words. The clincher was when I realized that I wouldn't be able to pass my annual CPR certification. I practiced at home on some stuffed animals just to be sure, but I got too winded and couldn't maintain the compressions.

So after 20 years, and catching over 3,000 babies, I had to retire at 55. It wasn't my plan, but whenever I catch myself feeling sorry or whiny, I remind myself that for 20 years I got to do something that I truly loved, that I felt called to do, and lots of people can't say that. Plus I had ten years before that working as a labor and delivery nurse, and another 4+ years in medical-surgery.

We've had events and situations in my family that might have been disastrous if I'd still been working, so I'm okay with it. This town is small enough that I run into people all the time — I either delivered their baby, their grandbaby, niece, whatever! They remember me and recognize me, so I know I've made a positive impact on this community. Everybody knows 'Rose'. I'm a one-name person, like Madonna or Cher!

I had short-term disability from my employer, and then eventually I was able to receive Social Security Disability from the U.S. federal government, as well as long-term employer disability. The employer disability will end soon when I turn 65, which will reduce my income by 50%. However, at that time I will be able to draw on my employee pension, which at this time is about half of the employer's disability. So that will bring me up to about 75% of my current income. But, I'm currently being taxed on the employer's disability, as well as some of the SSD, so I don't know how that will change with the pension. Since my income will be less, I'm hoping my taxes will be less.

Rose, 64, USA

I am totally disabled, and unable to work or study. Have broken my left leg two times. I've spent time in nursing homes. At one time I couldn't cook because I couldn't understand recipes. I worked in restaurants for over 20 years before. I have learned to use the computer, calculator and even the phone four different times. I lose all control of my numbers during bad times.

I have lost all of my friends except for one. Most of my family think I make things up. My husband almost left me at one time. We have now made it a point to go out at least once a week, and we are trying to make new friends.

I've been on disability since 1997. I've been audited twice, but have been told that they would be stopping the audit after I send in all of my paperwork.

Kathleen, 60, USA

Wow, this disease has affected our home life hugely, as I was the busy mum of five children, running around for them all, and doing everything in the household. And also working full time in a very senior position in a government department.

My husband has had to learn to cook, clean, run the household, grocery shop, menu plan, and so on.

Losing my income has had a huge impact as well. We can no longer keep our home and had to sell it, as we couldn't afford the mortgage anymore and also it was a two-storey house. We have recently moved to a smaller, single-level house.

It's been very hard on the kids, as they have to help me a lot around the house, and my youngest has had to help me when I have fallen over. When I'm too sick to get out of bed, he has had to make sure I have water, my drugs and so on my bedside for the day, before he goes to school. He also puts my shoes and socks on for me, as I cannot do this.

We now have no social life now really. We used to be quite the social couple and life of the party, but that was another person for me, as I just can't be bothered going out, or I am feeling too tired which is the main reason. Although we don't get asked anymore to go out — we have lost lots of friends because of this condition.

I don't think my friends realise how neurosarc has impacted me. I was always the organizer, and now I am not doing that, I just don't see anyone anymore. I only have a few friends, but I still don't think they really understand what I am going through. As you know, we often look well, and I think my friends only see that I have put on weight, and can't walk properly. And I must admit when I do see them, I do my makeup and hair, and do look well and laugh and joke with them, so they only see that part.

I can no longer work. I do not know how I will wake up each day. I can't retain any information, so would not be any good to anyone at this stage.

I cannot access any sort of disability pension or anything. I have tried through Centrelink, but because of my husband's income, we cannot get anything. We only just found out about Carer's Payment which my husband can get — it's $115 per fortnight. But that's it.

Jill, 51, Australia

Neurosarcoidosis affects every part of my life, but I try to not let it become my life. I cannot work any longer because I am too sick, and have way too many appointments. I also cannot have any children because of sarcoidosis. All of the medications at such a young age have made me infertile. My daily routine consist of lots of resting in between my daily chores, and taking lots of medication. I try to keep myself busy so that I do not become depressed. I have a lot of faith, and rely on God and my husband a lot to get me through the tough times.

I do not have a lot of friends that really come by or that I hang out with since I became sick. I don't really have a social life. My friends love and care about me, but I do not think they really get how serious this disease really is, because I look fine. I look like a normal 34 year old woman. Actually, I look about 23 which makes it worse, so I don't look sick at all.

I have been disabled since 25. I do attend online schooling through PennState. I am working on a Bachelor's in Letters, Arts and Sciences. I am a full time student which keeps my brain busy.

I have been able to receive Social Security since 2005, at the age of 27.

Andrea, 34, USA

Neurosarc has impacted my life tremendously!! I have always been extremely energetic in the past. I was one of those folks who would burn the candle at both ends. With my symptoms, I am unable to do the things that I would normally do. I cannot go hiking, I tire after being at a restaurant for a meal and get extremely restless, where I just want to go home. I have not been able to watch movies or TV because it makes me dizzy.

I live with my two dogs and cat. I was starting to feel a little depressed after being diagnosed and dealing with this by myself for five months, so I had my mother come to help me out. I was told not to drive, so felt further isolated and had trouble with doing errands such as groceries, going to the doctor appointments, and so on. I have trouble with fatigue, pain, shortness of breath and balance issues. She helps cook and take care of other odds and ends. I feel really awful that I am only 43, and my mother is in her late sixties, and she is taking care of me, where it should be the other way around...

I was told not to drive due to the dizziness, and cognitive fog, so that has been very stressful. I have to depend on friends to take or bring groceries for me, take me to doctor visits, my animals to the vet/pet store and so forth. They all have their busy lives, and often I would get frustrated, because sometimes they would say that they would come to help, and then never show up.

I have been really lucky, though, I do have a lot of friends in my support system, that have been my pillars. A few of them have disappeared, that I was really shocked about, because I was there for them when they were going through their difficult times. However, I have learned through this process that I should never expect anything from anyone. It makes me feel a lot happier. Several of my friends and co-workers have been very sympathetic towards my condition. Some of my younger friends, I believe, are uncomfortable with me being ill, and have not been in contact much.

The NS has profoundly affected my ability to work as a doctor. I have not been able to work for the last two years. I tried to do a half shift, yet because of the dyspnea, fatigue and arthralgias, I was not able to perform my basic duties at the hospital and the clinic. I have so much cognitive decline now that I am no longer able to practice medicine.

I had short term disability through my employer shortly after I was unable to work. This was switched to long-term disability, and I immediately qualified for Social Security Disability.

Dr Farah, 43, USA

I'm so exhausted all the time that I can't get out much to socialise. I do try to make the effort to see friends a few times a month, which often means they visit me at my home, or I sacrifice some of my energy to meet them at a café. I get quite sick if I go out at night, my pain levels increases a lot, and I'm really wiped out the next day.

My immediate family are wonderful. But they *all* have autoimmune diseases too (we're a bit 'special') so we really 'get' each other, as we're all in the same boat — but it also means we're all sick, all the time! This makes our family life difficult at times, and we don't get out much.

I think my extended family and friends try to understand. They don't think I'm making it up or anything like that. But they do forget at times, understandably. I've had to let go of some friendships with people who just didn't understand, and were too demanding. Other friends have faded away, when I stopped being the one who instigated our get-togethers.

I can still work, I run my own business from home, and I work nearly a full working week. I'm not well enough to work in an external office. I can't handle the commuting or being out that much in a day (I tried that a few years ago, put me into a relapse!).

I'm on some committees related to my book indexing profession, which add to my stress levels, but I'll be getting off them as soon as my current term is up. I try not to spend too much mental or emotional energy on them. I'm happy to do volunteer work, but my new 'maximum number of committees' will be **zero**!

My minor vision loss (which is right in the middle of my field of view, annoyingly) makes my work as an author, editor, and indexer a bit challenging at times, as I can sometimes miss seeing letters and details. I have to triple check my work. I don't read for pleasure much any more, as my eyes get too tired, dry and sore by the end of the day.

I sometimes find it harder to read and understand complicated books. My family says I get words wrong when I'm talking, and that my personality has changed a bit since I had my most severe sarc attack in 2010. I tend to be a bit more impulsive, and have more trouble concentrating.

I'm not eligible for any government support, because of my husband's income (which is average). My income from my business is very low, but it's better than doing nothing. It keeps me active, doing interesting things. But I know I'm unlikely to ever earn a full income.

Denise, 50, Australia

My neurosarc doesn't overly affect my home and family life. Since the diagnosis I feel pretty good, and I feel like I can manage it. My girlfriend and family have been fantastic, and in particular my mother and aunt.

My social life has been affected in that I find it difficult standing up for hours in a packed pub drinking pints and shots like I used to, LOL. I feel drinking makes my walk and balance much worse and unfortunately it's a big part of an Irish person's social life, and it's definitely something I have had to step back from. I don't think my friends understand it really, but I have some close friends that have been good and do look out for me.

Up until now it has affected my ability to work hugely. After I was discharged from hospital, I went on illness benefit which is more of a short term arrangement, and you are not allowed to work while receiving this. I applied for Disability Allowance in August 2012, which would enable me to work up to 20 hours per week while still receiving an allowance, and would also be supplied with a free travel pass enabling the bearer to free bus and rail travel all over Ireland.

Due to what I was told was a massive backlog of applicants, I did not get put on Disability Allowance until September 2013. I have applied for some jobs since being accepted but being a chef, it is harder to get work after the summer period, and it doesn't help when you have been out of employment for so long, and plus I'm only looking for part time work. I am eager to get back to work, as financially I am only just surviving at the moment.

Percy, 27, Ireland

I can no longer work, I'm mostly confined to wheelchair. I can use a walker now, but am not steady. I can no longer drive, go to the store to shop, travel, walk the dogs, exercise, go to activities at my son's school. My whole life has changed. EVERYTHING! I can't do anything I did before neurosarc without help now. I'm very limited in doing the things I try to do.

I have no social life. My marriage did not survive the illness. I don't like to go out for outings, because of the incontinence. I have good friends that stood by me, but I really don't think they understand how this has affected my life. Something as simple as a step up is impossible, or going into a crowded restaurant, people looking at you. It's just hard!

I am receiving Supplemental Security Income (SSI) Benefits. I have no health insurance or any other government assistance.

Linda, 49, USA

I had to stop working in the healthcare industry in 2005. My husband and I have two children. It's been extremely difficult. I can't stand to cook any more. I need help for even small things, like household chores, showering, and dressing. My husband, Russ, has had to take over.

He is what keeps me going. He makes me smile when I'm down, and gives up everything for our family. He has taken over so many roles and he never complains.

The hardest part was giving up my independence — working and driving a car. That was dreadfully hard. My dizziness is constant, so I use a walker all the time.

I am never left alone, because there's always the risk that I'll fall. My family and friends help out constantly, and look after me during the days when my husband is at work. I don't know what I'd do without them.

Kim, 48, USA

10
Coping strategies
and advice

In this chapter, I asked how do people cope with living with neurosarcoidosis, and what strategies help them. What sort of impact has neurosarc had on their psychological well-being. And finally, I asked what advice they'd give to people who are recently diagnosed.

I cope daily by spending time with my grandson who is now two — he reminds me of the blessings I have in my life. I love listening to my two adult children discuss current events. The doctors thought in 2006 I might not live. I am very much alive today — it is a struggle but I am doing it.

My hope, and the doctor's hope, is that I will go into remission. I keep hoping each day for some small sign that remission is around the corner. And of course I'm always hoping for a cure.

Kim, 48, USA

It could be worse. My faith and my beautiful eight grandchildren, who were born after I was diagnosed, help me to cope.

I have felt worthless. I strain on life. I hate to cry because then I get stuffed up. I have my pity parties once in a while (no one else is invited).

The fatigue is horrendous, learn to cope. Read everything you can. Talk to anyone you can. Pray and learn to laugh. I do love to laugh. Get dressed everyday. Put one foot in front of the other. Learn as much as you can and don't take no for an answer.

When a neurologist tells you it's all in your head prove to her that it is! If you're a doctor, don't make assumptions about your patients.

Kathleen, 60, USA

I feel I'm quite lucky with my neurosarc, I'm much less disabled than many. The relapsing-remitting type of NS is easier to live with. So I'm thankful for that. I'm pretty philosophical about the possibility of future disability — going blind is my biggest fear. I find my periodic loss of smell and taste quite distressing. I'm proactive about my health, and try my best to be as healthy as I can be within my limitations. I'm a client of Vision Australia, and other support networks, but don't need them at the moment.

I feel quite happy with what I've achieved in my professional life so far, so if I have to stop work at some point because of the neurosarc, I think I'll be okay about it. I'm well past the 'Why me' phase, and am resigned to my situation. It can all be very frustrating at times, though. I often do too much — I find pacing myself very hard. I'm slowly getting better at setting boundaries.

I do get depressed at times, and anxious. I tend to obsess and worry over new symptoms. Much of my anxiety is because I have 'medical PTSD' as a result of traumatic childhood surgeries (for hip dysplasia). My neurologist recently took the time to explain about functional neurological symptoms to me (see page 18), and this has really completely cured me of feeling anxious about new minor symptoms.

What helps me cope? A good sense of humour about everything, not taking myself seriously, the support, love and company of family and close friends, and my lovely dogs (best therapy ever). Swearing and the occasional rant helps too. I love drawing, painting, cooking and knitting, and do what I can within my limits (and sometimes outside of them!).

My advice for new neurosarcies? Firstly, it really sucks. Get proper medical treatment from proper doctors, and take the time to find specialists who know about neurosarc. Look for support groups online, and find others who are going through the same thing. Consider seeing a counsellor or psychologist.

Learn what you can about your disease (this book is a good start!). Try not to worry about 'little symptoms' too much. Read about the Spoon Theory. Live within your limits, but don't put your life on hold because of the neurosarc. Laugh a lot. Do things you love that you can still manage, drop the things you don't (although the dishes still need to be done — tragic, I know).

Stay in touch with the people who 'get it'. Know that some of your friends are fair weather friends, and they will abandon you. It hurts, but it's likely to happen and you need to let go of them. Learn about setting boundaries in your personal life, and work on it. Focus your energies on the people who support and love you.

Denise, 50, Australia

Something that helps me cope personally is health and fitness. Eating healthily was not something I was particularly interested in before I got neurosarc. It is something that I have developed an interest in hugely over the last year or so. I always had an interest in working out, but never had the drive to stick at it, and always gave up as soon as I had begun.

I feel like my experience with NS has made me grow up and mature as a person, and I am grateful for that. I can now stick at things more, and the healthy eating and fitness definitely helps psychologically — healthy body, healthy mind. I drink a green smoothie every day, and try to include as much fruits and vegetables in my diet as possible. I gained nearly 20 kilos (44 lb) from steroids — but I have now lost that extra weight, and I am now in good physical shape.

133

Psychologically it has been a very tough experience, but I really believe what doesn't kill you makes you stronger. And I think the fact that I fought through it and came out the other side is pretty cool.

The advice I would give is never let it get you down, take each challenge as it comes, be strong — knuckle down and get through it.

Percy, 27, Ireland

I try to keep a positive attitude. I go out everyday, regardless of how ill I am. Even if it is just sitting in the backyard. I exercise by taking my dogs out for walks. We may not be at the same pace as before, and take frequent breaks, but I try to get out twice a day for this.

This disease has had a profound effect on my emotions and psyche. I have always been a very high energy, positive, and active person. I dabbled in many things at the same time. My energy level and my memory were my super powers, and this disease has robbed me of them. It is extremely frustrating to want to do so many things, yet not being physically or mentally capable of it. I was an avid hiker before, and now get fatigued and short of breath with just walking the length of my house. I also enjoyed reading and writing, and now both of these skills have declined considerably. I have zero energy to travel, which is another one of my passions.

Being alone when I was first diagnosed and ill, I found that I had a lot of support from friends and family, however, as the disease is not responding to the usual regimen, and is lingering, it is amazing that several people have abandoned me. This has made me feel rather disheartened and sad. However, I have a few solid people that I can rely on, that makes my heart filled with gratitude.

The disease has affected my mental health in a way that I notice that I have become rather short-tempered and impatient with things. Perhaps, a component of this may be due to the medicines, and being in pain and so fatigued. I just notice that my personality has changed considerably with being ill. I am easily irritated. And often just speak my mind, whereas in the past, I would be polite and refrain from sharing my thoughts.

This disease is horrible, and can take away much of who you were and what you were capable of. Try to stay as positive as you can, although when there are bad days, you may have a harder time looking for things to be positive about. Also, try to keep up with some type of physical activity, no matter how mild. It will help. I definitely notice those two things make it much easier for me.

Dr Farah, 43, USA

What helps me cope? I pray a lot, and have a strong desire to walk. I work hard trying to stay positive.

For new patients, I recommend that you get a second opinion, ask lots of questions about the treatment plan, and have supportive people around.

I wished I had asked more questions when I was diagnosed with transverse myelitis. I think if my treatment plan had been better, I would not have had the second episode that left me paralysed.

Linda, 49, USA

I've always thought there were two options: to cope or not to cope. I chose to cope, but it's not without its challenges. I guess I've become very competitive within myself, like it's me versus the sarcoidosis. And if someone tells me I can't do something well, that just encourages me to do it. It can be hard not to get anxious about the disease — just when you think you are managing it, a new symptom or setback comes along, and you have to regroup and start all over again.

Getting NS in my 20s had a massive emotional impact on me. Especially as you watch your friends travel, have careers, marry, and have children. I have had a lot of counselling to learn to deal with it. I don't think you'd be human if it didn't upset you.

As horrible as having sarcoidosis is, I have met some lovely people who also have NS. My outlook on life has changed. I have been able to study and volunteer in areas I otherwise wouldn't have been able to. I think you have to make the best of what life throws at you.

I recommend you research the disease for yourself. Ask your doctors questions, and tell them if you're not coping. Take control of the management of the disease. Tap into the support groups online. The basic health advice we've always heard — eat well, exercise, rest — is beneficial. Laughter really can be good medicine. I also keep a journal (I'm up to the 5th one!) which helps to track what has been happening, but also allows me to get things off my chest.

Leah, 34, Australia

I use a combination of activity and rest throughout the day when I'm at my best. At my worst I will be in bed, almost hibernating till I improve. This can last for several months at a time. I shop online when possible. I do minimal housework and cooking, and socialise very little. My life is a mix of being too ill to be part of the human race, and being my optimistic happy self. When neurosarc dictates, I can't even contemplate a normal life so I don't miss it. At my best, I use every chance to live life and see friends and family.

I was brought up with the belief that if you can adapt to adversity, you'll always be okay. I've lowered my expectations and changed my aspirations. The brain issues cause a lack of confidence, in that I'm sometimes unsure of whether I'm remembering correctly. I'm so sorry I'm not the reliable person I should be. I have a natural resilience and use that to my advantage, but I'd rather I was achieving normal life goals, instead of overcoming the effects of NS.

Advice for new patients:

1) Join a support group; so many symptoms of neurosarc are not easily proven by medical tests so we're left with a negative frame of mind, and chatting with other sufferers gives affirmation.

2) Find out the possible effects so you don't hold back your symptoms at consultations. I've kept symptoms from doctors because I couldn't understand what was happening, and felt embarrassed, so I thought I wouldn't be believed.

3) Listen to your body, know your limits, and don't push yourself too hard.

4) Ask for help and share your plight with your family, they need to understand too.

As sarcoid is seen as an illness that mimics many other conditions, it isn't diagnosed until all other serious causes for symptoms are excluded, therefore it left me constantly feeling I'd failed each time I got that negative result.

It also means I've been left to suffer without treatment until the doctor has taken the time to rule out everything else. When a recent flare-up caused new neuro symptoms, my GP simply brushed it off saying that I am on the medication for NS and he knew from past experience that these episodes will pass! I'm in excruciating pain and he feels it's okay to ignore it, and just send me home with pain-killers.

I was due to see my neuro consultant and he cancelled, due to ill-health, so I asked my GP to refer me to a neuro consultant who is a specialist in NS. He has asked someone to see me, but this consultant has no record of NS as a specialty, so I'm having to ask again to be referred to Royal Free Hospital. It's been 20 months so far since I asked if he thought it could be NS. I feel so neglected and don't trust my GP now, as he's not listening to me.

Jacqui, 57, Scotland

Do you have a good support system through family and friends? Our personal relationships are impacted tremendously by any chronic illness, and neurosarc seems to be particularly nasty in that way. One of the problems for most of us is that it is an invisible disability. It's hard for family and friends to understand what's wrong with us, when in their eyes, we 'look so good!'

Remember that doctors (and nurses, etc.) work for you. If you are unsatisfied with any aspect of your care and cannot get it resolved, fire them and get somebody else. Most of us have a team of 'ologists' — regardless of where you are receiving care, you should feel confident, safe and respected by everyone on your medical team. Where are you being treated? Do you feel that your docs are up on current knowledge about sarcoidosis research and treatment options?

Keep notes of symptoms, things that worsen or improve the symptoms; drugs (prescription, OTC, supplements), and how they affect your symptoms or create new symptoms. Record all of your medical visits, with your questions and concerns, the results of that visit, other questions raised, and so on. Many like to use a notebook. I keep mine all on my computer (because I lose the notebooks, or the pencils), then I print out a copy for both the doc and me. Record even things that don't seem important. Then take this notebook to all of your appointments.

Also take an advocate to your medical appointments. Could be a husband, adult child, friend (I took my pastor's wife once!). They do not need a medical background, but they need to be assertive (not aggressive) and willing to stand up for you. Give the advocate a copy of your questions for that visit, and their job is to stand in front of the door, and not let the doctor leave that room until you are satisfied with the discussion and plan.

When a test or drug is suggested, ask what are the potential benefits and possible side effects or complications. Regarding tests, ask if the result changes the treatment plan. You should have input into the treatment plan, after weighing the possible benefits vs.

risks. For example, after two discussions with my cardiologist/
electrophysiologist and research on my own, I opted for the AICD for
my cardiac sarc, even though that eliminates future MRIs. But it was
an informed decision.

It's common for a person with one immune disorder to develop
others (such as rheumatoid arthritis). This can definitely complicate
the diagnostic process. NS is tricky because there isn't a test that says,
yep, that's it. If you have biopsy-confirmed sarc and then develop
neurologic symptoms, NS is a fairly likely culprit, although other
causes still need to be ruled out.

However, there are a number of folks who only have neurologic
symptoms and no sarc on biopsy. For those people, the diagnosis has
been made (or presumed enough to warrant treatment) by a physician
skilled and experienced enough to combine the health history,
comprehensive physical exam (with a detailed neuro exam, not done
by most docs), and any pertinent lab/procedure results. **These docs are
rare birds, but they're out there.**

Sometimes we get lucky right off the bat, most times we have to be
persistent and assertive. You may need someone to fill that role, or
at least help you. This can involve a lot of online research, looking
for docs with the expertise needed, even traveling a distance to
see these docs. Many of us have had to educate our docs; some of
them welcome the input and others do not. It can be discouraging,
infuriating, exhausting, but also empowering.

Rose, 64, USA

Neurosarc has changed me. I am a more caring and empathetic person
now. I really value life and all it has to offer. I have hit rock bottom a
few time with sarcoidosis, and I have almost died from this disease. It
can be very taxing on your emotions — one minute you're anxious and
worried, and the next minute you're depressed.

I pray a lot, my faith in God is the number one thing, and my husband. I also enjoy planting and growing things and crafting in general. I am a hands-on person.

Never give up and never let anyone make you feel like your symptoms aren't real, because they are. Don't stop trying to get someone to listen to you. Eventually there will be someone who knows what you're going through, you just have to find them.

Andrea, 34, USA

I just live day to day, as I never know how I am going to wake up each day. I have my laptop computer that I love, and would be very lost without it every day, as I am on it all the time.

I have taught myself to crochet. I did this because I thought I was having a lot of trouble reading and remembering anything at all. So I watched YouTube videos. It was very hard to read a line of a pattern, then put it into practice. I have been crocheting for one year now, but still feel I am a beginner, as I can't remember anything from the last year. It's frustrating as other people think that I should know more, but I still can't retain anything!

I am a positive person usually, so still try to be that — but at times it can be very hard to do.

I was more upset when I got the blood clot than when I was told I had two months to live (from an incorrect brain cancer diagnosis)! This was because my father had a blood clot in the same spot and it travelled up thru his heart and killed him. It was only then that I realised just how severe this condition was!

The other time I was quite sad is when I have had my driver's license suspended. I know I can't drive anymore, but the fact that I don't have a license has been very upsetting and it is like 'This is just another thing this bloody disease has taken off me!'

140

Advice:

Do some research of your own. You can learn a lot from other support groups. I saved my eyesight using that group, and reading people's blogs and posts.

I feel very isolated. Nobody knows or understands my condition, as much as I try and put it out there. If only I had MS — people seem to know what that's all about, and have a better understanding.

There are no sarcoidosis support groups around me — so that's why I belong to them on Facebook — well worth it.

Jill, 51, Australia

Afterword

So, here we are at the end of the book. As you can see, neurosarcoidosis can be a very challenging disease to live with, whether you have it yourself, or someone you love has it.

Research into this disease is still rather thin on the ground. Getting a clear diagnosis is extremely difficult, treatments can be a bit hit or miss, and medications often have significant side effects.

Despite these difficulties, us neurosarcies live our lives as best we can, and don't give in to the disease. We do our best to be advocates for our own health, raising awareness and knowledge of the disease when we can, struggling onwards, trying to live within the limitations imposed by the disease, and often still caring for family, and attempting to work or study as well.

Yes, we're doing it tough, but *we're* tough.

We're pretty damn awesome.

Further reading

Books

Bright-sided: How Positive Thinking is Undermining America, B. Ehrenreich

Coping with Prednisone, Dr J. Ingelfinger and E. Zuckerman

Navigating Smell and Taste Disorders, R. DeVere MD and M. Calvert

Sick and Tired of Feeling Sick and Tired, P. Donoghue and M. Siegel

Trick or Treatment, S. Singh and E. Ernst

Websites

Medical information

Choosing Wisely — American Board of Internal Medicine
Very useful set of lists to help make medical decisions
www.choosingwisely.org/doctor-patient-lists/

Drugs.com
www.drugs.com

The Foundation for Peripheral Neuropathy
www.foundationforpn.org

Foundation for Sarcoidosis Research
www.stopsarcoidosis.org

Functional and Dissociative Neurological Symptoms
www.neurosymptoms.org

Health Central
www.healthcentral.com

Lab Tests Online
labtestsonline.org

PsychCentral
Search for articles on chronic illness, setting boundaries etc.
psychcentral.com

Quackwatch
www.quackwatch.com

Science Based Medicine blog
www.sciencebasedmedicine.org

Sense About Science
www.senseaboutscience.org

WebMD
www.webmd.com

Diet and Lifestyle

Art Therapy blog
www.arttherapyblog.com

Fast Day
www.fastday.com

The Fast Diet
thefastdiet.co.uk

MyFitnessPal
www.myfitnesspal.com

Support groups and organisations

But you don't look sick
www.butyoudontlooksick.com

Facebook: Neurosarcoidosis group
www.facebook.com/groups/7337716399/

Fifth Sense (loss of smell & taste)
www.fifthsense.org.uk

Living with Facial Paralysis
www.facialnervepalsy.com

National Sarcoidosis Organization (Canada)
www.nationalsarcoidosisorganization.com

The Neurological Alliance
www.neural.org.uk

The Neuropathy Association
www.neuropathy.org

Yahoo email list — Neurosarcoidosis
groups.yahoo.com/neo/groups/neurosarcoidosis/info

Rare Voices Australia
www.rarevoices.org.au

Disability rights

Americans with Disability Act
www.ada.gov

Australian Human Rights Commission
Search for disability rights
www.humanrights.gov.au

Disability Rights UK
disabilityrightsuk.org

Disability rights – GOV.UK
www.gov.uk/browse/disabilities/rights

Abbreviations

ACE .... angiotensin converting enzyme
ANA .... anti-nuclear antibody
BAL .... bronchoalveolar lavage
CNS .... central nervous system
CRP .... C-reactive protein
CT .... computed tomography
EEG .... electroencephalogram, scan that records electrical activity of the brain
EMG .... electromyogram, scan that records electrical activity of muscles and motor nerves
ENT .... ear, nose and throat
ER .... emergency room
ESR .... erythrocyte sedimentation rate
FBC .... full blood count
GI .... glycaemic index
GP .... general practitioner
IUD .... intrauterine device
IV .... intravenous
IVIG .... intravenous immunoglobulin
LP .... lumbar puncture
MRI .... magnetic resonance imaging
MS .... multiple sclerosis
NS .... neurosarcoidosis
OTC .... over the counter
PCP .... primary care physician
PET .... positron emission tomography
PNS .... peripheral nervous system
PTSD .... post traumatic stress disorder
Q-SART .... quantitative sudomotor axon reflex test
SPF .... sun protection factor
TENS .... transcutaneous electrical nerve stimulation
TNF .... tumor necrosis factor
UTI .... urinary tract infection
VER .... visual evoked potential

Glossary

acetylcholine — a neurotransmitter molecule; sends signals from one nerve cell to another

acute — severe, but only lasting a short time

adipocyte — fat cell

adipokine — cell signalling molecule secreted by fat cells

adrenal cortex — outer layer of the adrenal gland; it produces corticosteroids, cortisol, and other hormones like testosterone

adrenal crisis — deadly situation from a sudden deficiency of cortisol, which can be caused by suddenly stopping corticosteroids

aetiology — cause of a disease

allogenic — tissues or cells donated from another person

anaemic — suffering from anaemia, a red blood cell or iron deficiency

angiogram — x-ray image of blood or lymph vessels, involving the injection of a contrast agent via femoral catheter

antacid — substance that neutralises stomach acidity

antigen — substance which causes an immune response in the body

aphasia — language disorder caused by brain damage; can involve loss of ability to speak, read, or write

arrhythmia — irregular heart beat

arthralgia — joint pain

asbestosis — lung disease from inhalation of asbestos fibres

aseptic — free from contamination by bacteria, viruses etc

atrial fibrillation — common type of abnormal heart rhythm

atrophy — waste away

autonomic — involuntary or unconscious

autonomic nervous system — nerves responsible for controlling unconscious body functions, such as breathing, beating of the heart, and digestion

Behcet's disease — systemic small blood vessel vasculitis

bilateral — affecting both sides of the body

biopsy — examination of a tissue sample to discover the type, cause or extent of a disease

bronchoscope — a thin flexible fibre optic instrument used to get tissue samples from the lungs, and look inside the lungs

147

cachexin / cachectin — tumor necrosis factor

calcitriol — hormonally active form of vitamin D, that increases blood calcium levels

cannula — very thin tube inserted into a vein for delivery of fluids, medications, or a surgical instrument

caseation — turning into a cheese-like mass of diseased tissue

cataract — opaque clouding of the eye lens, leading to blindness

cat scratch disease — infectious disease caused by bacteria introduced into the body by the scratch or bite of a cat

catheter — thin tube inserted into the body for delivery of fluids or gases, for access for surgical instruments, or to allow drainage

CellCept — brand name for mycophenolate mofetil, an immune suppressant

central nervous system — brain and spinal cord

chronic — lasting for a long time, or constantly recurring

circadian rhythm — any biological cycle that recurs on a roughly 24 hour cycle

collagen — structural protein in connective tissue

connective tissue — tissue that connects, supports, binds, or separates other tissues or organs from each other

contagious — liable to be transmitted to others through direct contact

contrast agent — substance used to enhance the visualisation of body structures or fluids during medical imaging

convulsion — fit caused by abnormal electric activity in the brain

corticosteroids — steroid hormones that are produced naturally in the body, as well as being produced as medicines

cortisol — a steroid hormone released by the adrenal cortices

cranium — the upper part of the skull, separate from the jawbone

Crohn's disease — chronic inflammatory disease of the intestine

delusion — belief held despite contradiction with reality or logic

dermatologist — a skin specialist

dopamine — hormone and neurotransmitter

dysautonomia — malfunctioning of the autonomic nervous system

dyscalculia — difficulty understanding numbers and arithmetic

dysesthesia — neurological disorder with abnormal and unpleasant sense of touch, typically presenting as pain

dyspnea —shortness of breath

electrolyte — a substance (like salt) that ionises (gets a negative or positive charge) when dissolved in a solvent such as water

electrophysiologist — doctor who studies the electrical properties of biological cells and tissues

erythrocyte — red blood cell

fibroblast — cell in connective tissue that produces collagen and other fibres

fluoroscopy — live action x-ray imaging technique, used during medical procedures to guide the doctor

folic acid — an essential B vitamin that helps the body to create and repair DNA, and produce new red blood cells

glaucoma — eye disorder resulting in optic nerve damage and vision loss, caused by high pressure inside the eye

glycaemic index — number associated with how quickly a particular food is digested, and how it affects blood sugar

granuloma — small lump of tissue

granulomatous — causing formation of granulomas

haemoglobin — iron-containing protein that carries oxygen in red blood cells

hepatologist — a liver specialist

hilar nodes — lymph nodes in the lungs

histoplasmosis — fungal infection found in bat and bird droppings, not serious if only affecting the lungs; can be fatal if spread through the body

hypercalcaemia — high levels of calcium in the blood

hydrocephalus — accumulation of fluid within the brain

hypotension — low blood pressure

hypothalamus — part of the brain that coordinates the autonomic nervous system

immunologist — an immune system specialist

immunoglobulin — another name for an antibody; a protein that identifies and neutralises foreign particles in the body

Imuran — brand name for azathioprine

incidence — occurrence, rate, or frequency of a disease

infectious — liable to be transmitted to others through the environment

infusion — the introduction of a drug or fluid into the body via IV

jaundice — yellow pigmentation of the skin from high levels of bilirubin in the body, caused by liver disease

leptomeninges — the lower two layers of membranes covering the brain (pia mater and arachnoid layer), viewed as a single layer

leprosy — contagious bacterial disease that affects the skin, mucous membranes and nerves

lesion — area in an organ or tissue that has been damaged by injury or disease

leucocyte — white blood cell

lupus — systemic autoimmune disease

Lyme disease — infectious disease caused by bacteria, transferred by tick bite

lymph — colourless fluid containing white blood cells, which bathes tissues

lymphadenopathy — disease affecting the lymph nodes

lymphatic system — network of vessels through body which lymph drains from the tissues into the blood

lymph nodes — nodes in body where lymph is filtered and lymphocytes are formed

lymphocyte — small white blood cell, found in the lymphatic system

lymphoma — blood cell tumor that develops from lymphocytes

macrophage — white cell that engulfs bacteria and particles

mediastinoscopy — scope procedure that looks inside the chest cavity (but not inside the lungs)

Ménière's disease — disorder of the inner ear, affecting hearing and balance

meninges — three membranes that line the skull and vertebral column, and cover the brain and spinal cord

meningitis — inflammation of the meninges, the membranes covering the brain

metabolism — chemical reactions that happen inside the body to sustain life, typically breaking down food to create energy, creating proteins etc.

methemoglobinemia — a blood disorder that leads to less oxygen in the body

multiple sclerosis — autoimmune disease causing progressive damage to nerve cell sheaths

mycobacterium — bacterium of a group that includes those that cause leprosy and tuberculosis

myelopathy — disease of the spinal cord

myopathy — disease of muscle tissue

neuralgia — nerve pain

neurologist — a nerve specialist

neuropathologist — pathologist who studies nervous system tissues

neuropathy — disease or dysfunction of the nerves

neuropsychiatry — psychiatry relating to mental or emotional problems caused by disordered brain function

non-caseating — not developing into cheese-like mass of diseased tissue; containing live cells

non-invasive — not using medical instruments inserted into the body

non-necrotising — not dying; alive

nonspecific — not assigned to a particular cause or disease

oligoclonal bands — bands of antibodies that appear in certain positions on an electrophoresis gel testing cerebrospinal fluid or blood serum; they are indicative of antibodies and therefore disease processes in the central nervous system

onycholysis — condition where the nail painlessly separates from the nail bed

optic neuritis — inflammation of the optic nerve

optic chiasm — X-shaped structure where the two optic nerves cross over each other, under the brain

orthopaedic — relating to deformities of the bones and muscles

osteoporosis — brittle and fragile bones from loss of tissue, generally as a result of calcium and vitamin D deficiency

oxytocin — hormone that acts as a neuromodulator in the brain and is involved in childbirth, breastfeeding, and bonding

palsy — paralysis, especially the kind with involuntary tremors

parenchyma — the grey matter of the brain, containing all the functional nerves

paraesthesia — tingling, burning, pins and needles, and other abnormal sensations, caused by damage to the peripheral nerves

parasomnias — group of sleep disorders that involve abnormal movements, perceptions, behaviours etc at various sleep stages, including sleep walking and restless legs syndrome

paroxysmal nocturnal dyspnea — attacks of severe shortness of breath and coughing that occur at night

pathologist — doctor who studies the causes of diseases, and analyses blood and other tests

peripheral nervous system — all the nerves outside of the central nervous system

peripheral neuropathy — disease or dysfunction of the peripheral nerves

pituitary gland — gland at the base of the hypothalamus that excretes hormones

plasmapheresis — removal, treatment, and return of blood plasma, removing autoantibodies from the blood system

platelets — blood cells that stop bleeding by clumping and clotting

prednisolone — corticosteroid medication

prognosis — likely course of a disease

progression — worsening of a disease

psychosis — severe mental disorder causing loss of connection to reality

pulmonary — relating to the lungs

pulmonary embolism — blood clot that blocks an artery in the lungs

remission — temporary reduction of severity of a disease

relapsing-remitting — disease that has flares interspersed with periods of low disease activity

rheumatoid arthritis — chronic progressive disease affecting the joints

scotoma — patch of low vision in the field of view

sedative — medicine that has a calming or tranquillising effect

sensory deficit — defect in the function of one of the senses (sight, hearing, taste, smell, touch)

seizure — fit caused by abnormal electric activity in the brain

septic — infected with bacteria

shunt — surgically-inserted thin tube to provide an alternative path for the passage of blood or other body fluid

Sjögren's syndrome — autoimmune disorder where white blood cells attacks the salivary and tear glands, leading to dryness

small fibre neuropathy — disease or dysfunction of the small peripheral nerve fibres

steroid-sparing agent — medication that allows a lower dose of steroid medication, or none, to be used, for a similar effect

stroma — non-nervous tissues of the brain: connective tissues, blood vessels etc

subcutaneous — under the skin

systemic — affecting the whole body

T-cell — T-lymphocyte, a type of white blood cell

transverse myelitis — inflammation of the spinal cord, causing loss of the myelin sheath of nerve fibres

trigeminal nerve — largest cranial nerve, responsible for sensation in the face and motor functions (e.g. biting and chewing)

tuberculosis — infectious bacterial disease, mainly affecting the lungs

tumor necrosis factor — a molecule that regulates immune cells

unilateral — affecting one side of the body

uvea — pigmented area of the eye

uveitis — inflammation of the uvea

vasculitis — inflammation of blood vessels

ventricle — hollow part in an organ, esp in the heart, or one of the four fluid-filled cavities in the middle of the brain

Wegener's granulomatosis — form of vasculitis, with formation of granulomas and inflammation of blood vessels. Also called granulomatosis with polyangiitis (GPA).

References

1. Nozaki, K and Judson, MA, 'Neurosarcoidosis: Clinical manifestations, diagnosis and treatment', *Presse Med.* 2012; 41: e331–e348

2. Bucurescu, G et al, *Neurosarcoidosis,* Medscape Reference, 2013, emedicine.medscape.com/article/1147324-overview, accessed Sept 2013

3. Iannuzzi, MC, Rybicki, BA, and Teirstein, AS, 'Sarcoidosis', *N Engl J Med.* 2007; 357: 2153–2165

4. Gillman, A and Steinfort, C. 'Sarcoidosis in Australia', *Intern Med J.* 2007 Jun; 37(6): 356–9

5. Hoitsma, E and Sharma, OP, 'Neurosarcoidosis', Chapter 11, in *Sarcoidosis,* edited by Drent, M and Costabel, U., European Respiratory Monograph, 2005 Sept, Vol 10, Monograph 32, pp 164–187

6. Nozaki, K and Judson, MA, 'Neurosarcoidosis', *Current Treatment Options in Neurology,* Neurologic Manifestations of Systemic Disease, ed Priutt, A., Springer Science+Business Media, New York, 2013

7. Dutra, LA et al, 'Neurosarcoidosis: Guidance for the general neurologist', *Arq Neuropsiquiatr.* 2012 Apr; 70(4): 293–299

8. Spiegel, DR, Morris, K, and Rayamajhi, U, 'Neurosarcoidosis and the Complexity in its Differential Diagnosis', *Innovations in Clinical Neuroscience*, 2012, Vol 9, No 4, 10–16

9. Oswald-Richter, KA et al. 'Dual analysis for mycobacteria and propionibacteria in sarcoidosis BAL', *J Clin Immunol,* 2012 Oct; 32(5): 1129–40

10. Drake, WP et al. 'Molecular Analysis of Sarcoidosis Tissues for Mycobacterium Species DNA', *Emerg Infect Dis* [serial online] 2002 Nov. Available from wwwnc.cdc.gov/eid/article/8/11/02-0318.htm. Accessed July 2013.

11. Thomeer, M et al, 'Epidemiology of sarcoidosis', Chapter 2 in *Sarcoidosis,* edited by Drent, M and Costabel, U., European Respiratory Monograph, 2005 Sept, Vol 10, Monograph 32, pp 13-22

12. Pardo, C, 'Neurosarcoidosis: Clinical, Pathological and Therapeutic Issues', *Transverse Myelitis Association*, Journal Vol 5, Jan 2011

13. Scott, TF et al, 'Aggressive Therapy for Neurosarcoidosis – Long-term Follow-up of 48 Treated Patients', *Arch Neurol.* 2007; 64: 691–696

14. Segal, BM, 'Neurosarcoidosis: diagnostic approaches and therapeutic strategies', *Curr Opin Neurol*, 2013 June; 26(3): 307–13

15. Zuckerman, E and Ingelfinger, J, *Coping with Prednisone*, St. Martin's Griffin, New York, 2007

16. Crislip, M, 'The Marshall Protocol' (17 July 2009) and 'The Microbial Metagenome' (14 August 2009), *Science–Based Medicine*, www.sciencebasedmedicine.org/the-marshal-protocol/ and www.sciencebasedmedicine.org/the-microbial-metagenome/, accessed January 2015

17. Pawate, HM and Sriram, S, 'Presentation and outcomes of neurosarcoidosis: a study of 54 cases', *Q J Med.* 2009; 102: 449–460

18. CellCept medication information, side effects: www.drugs.com/sfx/cellcept-side-effects.html, accessed September 2013

19. *Non-melanoma skin cancer: General practice consultation, hospitalisation and mortality*, Australian Institute of Health and Welfare and Cancer Australia, Sept 2008

20. Finlayson, G et al, 'Acute compensatory eating following exercise is associated with implicit hedonic wanting for food', *Physiol Behav.* 2009 Apr 20; 97(1): 62–7

21. Gleim, GW, 'Exercise is not an effective weight loss modality in women', *J Am Coll Nutr.* 1993 Aug; 12(4): 363–7.

22. Bacon, L, *Healthy at Every Size*, BenBella Books, 2010, pp 51–54

23. Cleveland Clinic, *Sarcoidosis Treatment Options*, my.clevelandclinic.org/disorders/sarcoidosis/hic_sarcoidosis_treatment_options.aspx, accessed Sept 2013

24. Baughman, RP and Lower, EE, 'Therapy for sarcoidosis', Chapter 20 in *Sarcoidosis*, edited by Drent, M and Costabel, U., European Respiratory Monograph, 2005 Sept, Vol 10, Monograph 32, 301–315

25. Hostettler, KE et al, 'Long-term treatment with infliximab in patients with sarcoidosis', *Respiration*, 2012; 83(3): 218–224

26. Chintamaneni, S et al, 'Dramatic response to infliximab in refractory neurosarcoidosis', *Ann Indian Acad Neurol*. 2010 Jul-Sep; 13(3): 207–210

27. 'Sarcoidosis Causes', News-Medical.net, www.news-medical.net/health/Sarcoidosis-Causes.aspx, accessed Sept 2013

28. 'Sarcoidosis', Epilepsy.com, professionals.epilepsy.com/page/inflammatory_sardcoidosis.html, accessed Oct 2013

29. 'Radiation Dose in X-ray and CT Exams', RadiologyInfo.org, www.radiologyinfo.org/en/safety/?pg=sfty_xray, accessed Oct 2013

30. *Information about radiation from diagnostic imaging procedures*, Environmental Health and Safety Program, University of Pennsylvania, www.ehrs.upenn.edu/media_files/docs/pdf/websiteinfo(2).pdf, accessed Oct 2013

31. 'Lumbar puncture', WebMD, www.webmd.com/brain/lumbar-puncture, accessed Oct 2013

32. Ehrenreich, B, *Bright–Sided: How positive thinking is undermining America*, Picador, 2009, pp 162–166

33. Smyth JM, Stone AA, Hurewitz A, Kaell A, 'Effects of Writing About Stressful Experiences on Symptom Reduction in Patients With Asthma or Rheumatoid Arthritis : A Randomized Trial', *The Journal of the American Medical Association*, 1999;281(14):1304-1309. doi: 10.1001/jama.281.14.1304.

34. Baikie KA, Kay Wilhelm K, 'Emotional and physical health benefits of expressive writing', *Advances in Psychiatric Treatment*, (2005) 11: 338-346

35. Crislip, M, 'Herbal "Remedies". Like "Fresh" Fish.' *Quackcast*, Episode 13, 22 January 2007 edgydoc.com/references/

36. 'The healing power of do-it-yourself music therapy', Bottom Line Publications, 19 August 2010, www.bottomlinepublications.com/content/article/self-improvement/the-healing-power-of-do-it-yourself-music-therapy, accessed Dec 2014

INDEX

Patient story references indicate more significant mentions in the text.